T0192375

SpringerBriefs in Statistics

JSS Research Series in Statistics

The current research of statistics in Japan has expanded in several directions in line with recent trends in academic activities in the area of statistics and statistical sciences over the globe. The core of these research activities in statistics in Japan has been the Japan Statistical Society (JSS). This society, the oldest and largest academic organization for statistics in Japan, was founded in 1931 by a handful of pioneer statisticians and economists and now has a history of about 80 years. Many distinguished scholars have been members, including the influential statistician Hirotugu Akaike, who was a past president of JSS, and the notable mathematician Kiyosi Itô, who was an earlier member of the Institute of Statistical Mathematics (ISM), which has been a closely related organization since the establishment of ISM. The society has two academic journals: the Journal of the Japan Statistical Society (English Series) and the Journal of the Japan Statistical Society (Japanese Series). The membership of JSS consists of researchers, teachers, and professional statisticians in many different fields including mathematics, statistics, engineering, medical sciences, government statistics, economics, business, psychology, education, and many other natural, biological, and social sciences. The JSS Series of Statistics aims to publish recent results of current research activities in the areas of statistics and statistical sciences in Japan that otherwise would not be available in English; they are complementary to the two JSS academic journals, both English and Japanese. Because the scope of a research paper in academic journals inevitably has become narrowly focused and condensed in recent years, this series is intended to fill the gap between academic research activities and the form of a single academic paper. The series will be of great interest to a wide audience of researchers, teachers, professional statisticians, and graduate students in many countries who are interested in statistics and statistical sciences, in statistical theory, and in various areas of statistical applications.

More information about this subseries at http://www.springer.com/series/13497

Hisayuki Tsukuma · Tatsuya Kubokawa

Shrinkage Estimation for Mean and Covariance Matrices

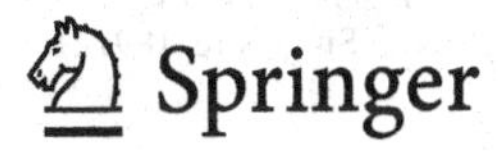
Springer

Hisayuki Tsukuma
Faculty of Medicine
Toho University
Tokyo, Japan

Tatsuya Kubokawa
Faculty of Economics
University of Tokyo
Tokyo, Japan

ISSN 2191-544X ISSN 2191-5458 (electronic)
SpringerBriefs in Statistics
ISSN 2364-0057 ISSN 2364-0065 (electronic)
JSS Research Series in Statistics
ISBN 978-981-15-1595-8 ISBN 978-981-15-1596-5 (eBook)
https://doi.org/10.1007/978-981-15-1596-5

This Springer imprint is published by the registered company Springer Nature Singapore Pte Ltd.
The registered company address is: 152 Beach Road, #21-01/04 Gateway East, Singapore 189721, Singapore

Preface

The rapid development of computer technology has started to yield many types of high-dimensional data and to enable us to deal with them well. Indeed, high-dimensional data appear in numerous fields such as web data science, genomics, telecommunication, atmospheric science, financial engineering, and others. With such a background, theory of statistical inference with high dimension has received much attention in recent years.

High-dimensional data in general are hard to handle, and ordinary or traditional methods in statistics are frequently inapplicable for them. This has inspired statisticians to develop new methodology in high dimension from both theoretical and practical aspects. Most statisticians' interests seem to be in development of efficient algorithms for statistical inference and in investigation of their asymptotic properties with the dimension going to infinity. On the other hand, there does not exist much literature in high-dimensional problems from a decision-theoretic point of view.

Statistical decision theory is the study of how to make decisions in the presence of statistical knowledge under uncertainty. It has been studied from around the 1940s and the researchers have already been produced many important and interesting results. Probably the most surprising result in decision-theoretic estimation is the inadmissibility of the sample mean vector to estimate a multivariate normal population mean. In the multivariate normal mean estimation, the sample mean vector is the maximum likelihood estimator and the uniformly minimum variance unbiased estimator, and thus it has been recognized to be optimal for a long time. However, in 1956, Charles Stein showed that the sample mean vector is admissible for the one- and two-dimensional cases but inadmissible for three or more dimensional cases. A little after that, a specific estimator, called a shrinkage estimator, was provided for exactly dominating the sample mean vector. To this day, various extensions of shrinkage estimation have been achieving in other statistical models.

The purpose of this book is to give a brief overview of shrinkage estimation in matrix-variate normal distribution model. More specifically, it includes recent techniques and results in estimation of mean and covariance matrices with a high-dimensional setting that implies singularity of the sample covariance matrix. Such a high-dimensional model can really be analyzed by using the same arguments as for a low-dimensional model. Thus this book takes a unified approach to both high- and low-dimensional shrinkage estimation.

Theory of shrinkage estimation for matrix parameters needs many mathematical tools. In Chap. 1, we begin by briefly introducing basic terminology of decision-theoretic estimation and a mathematical technique in shrinkage estimation. Chapter 2 defines the notation with respect to matrix algebra and collects useful results in terms of the Moore-Penrose inverse, the Kronecker product and matrix decompositions. Chapter 3 provides the definition and some properties of matrix-variate normal distribution and related distributions, including the Wishart distribution and joint distributions corresponding to the Cholesky and the eigenvalue decompositions of the Wishart matrix. With a unified treatment for high- and low-dimensional cases, some related distributions are discussed. Chapter 4 introduces a multivariate linear model and derives its canonical form. To find decision-theoretically optimal estimators, we usually direct our attention to several classes of invariant estimators. Therefore Chap. 4 briefly explains group invariance in the canonical form as well. A key tool in shrinkage estimation is an integration by parts formula, called the Stein identity. Chapter 5 gives a generalized Stein identity on matrix-variate normal distribution. Moreover we list some results on matrix differential operators and in particular show useful differentiation formulae concerning the Moore-Penrose inverse. Chapter 6 addresses the problem of estimating the mean matrix in matrix-variate normal distribution model. A unified result on matricial shrinkage estimation is presented, and extensions and applications are given for more general models. Chapter 7 deals with the problem of estimating the covariance matrix relative to an extended Stein loss and provides various unified estimation procedures for high- and low-dimensional cases. Some related topics to covariance estimation are also touched.

The authors would like to thank Prof. M. Akahira for giving us the opportunity of publishing this book. The work of the first author was supported in part by Grant-in-Aid for Scientific Research (18K11201) from the Japan Society for the Promotion of Science (JSPI). The work of the second author was supported in part by Grant-in-Aid for Scientific Research (18K11188) from the JSPI.

Tokyo, Japan
March 2020

Hisayuki Tsukuma
Tatsuya Kubokawa

Contents

Chapter 1
Decision-Theoretic Approach to Estimation

Statistical decision theory has been studied from around the 1940s and the researchers have already been producing many remarkable results. In the field of decision-theoretic estimation, the most surprising result is the inadmissibility of the sample mean vector in estimation of a mean vector of multivariate normal distribution. The inadmissibility result is closely relevant to the discovery of shrinkage estimator. This chapter summarizes basic terminology of decision-theoretic estimation and shrinkage estimators in the multivariate normal mean estimation. Also, Stein's unbiased estimate of risk is briefly explained as a general method of how to find better estimators. The unbiased risk estimate method is applied to estimation of mean and covariance matrices discussed in this book.

1.1 Decision-Theoretic Framework for Estimation

Let x be a random vector or matrix having a probability distribution characterized by an unknown parameter θ (possibly, θ can be a vector or matrix). Assume that we want to estimate θ based on x. An estimator of θ is denoted by $\hat{\theta} = \hat{\theta}(x)$ which is a function of x. In the literature $\hat{\theta}$ is also called the decision rule.

Let $\mathcal{P}$ be the parameter space. There are usually many estimation procedures for the unknown parameter $\theta \in \mathcal{P}$ and thus we need to decide how to select an optimal procedure. From an intuitive point of view, it seems reasonable to select an estimator minimizing a mathematical distance between $\hat{\theta}$ and θ or making it smaller as soon as possible. In statistical decision theory, such a distance is regarded as the loss induced from $\hat{\theta}$ by estimating θ. For this reason, the distance is called a loss function of $\hat{\theta}$ and θ. The loss function of $\hat{\theta}$ and θ is denoted by $L(\hat{\theta}, \theta)$, where it is nonnegative for any $\hat{\theta}$ and θ. We usually employ a loss function with properties that it takes zero when $\hat{\theta}$ is equal to θ and increases when $\hat{\theta}$ goes away from θ.

H. Tsukuma and T. Kubokawa, *Shrinkage Estimation for Mean and Covariance Matrices*,
JSS Research Series in Statistics, https://doi.org/10.1007/978-981-15-1596-5_1

However, the loss function of $\hat{\theta}$ and θ is random, and practically a distance between $\hat{\theta}$ and θ is measured by an expected loss

$$R(\hat{\theta}, \theta) = E[L(\hat{\theta}, \theta)],$$

where E denotes the expectation taken with respect to the distribution of x. Here $R(\hat{\theta}, \theta)$ is viewed as a quantified risk induced from $\hat{\theta}$ by estimating θ and it is called the risk function relative to $L(\hat{\theta}, \theta)$.

The risk function evaluates performance of estimators and can be employed to compare two estimators. If

$$R(\hat{\theta}_0, \theta) \leq R(\hat{\theta}, \theta)$$

for any $\theta \in \mathcal{P}$, with strict inequality for some θ, then an estimator $\hat{\theta}_0$ is said to be better than $\hat{\theta}$, or dominate $\hat{\theta}$, or improve on $\hat{\theta}$. An estimator $\hat{\theta}$ is said to be inadmissible if there exists another estimator $\hat{\theta}_0$ which dominates $\hat{\theta}$ and to be admissible if no such estimator $\hat{\theta}_0$ exists. For example, if we want to prove inadmissibility of an estimator then it simply suffices to find another dominating estimator.

Admissibility is a fundamental criterion in decision-theoretic estimation, but in general there exist many admissible estimators. Therefore we consider another criterion called minimaxity. The minimaxity of an estimator $\hat{\theta}_0$ implies that $\hat{\theta}_0$ minimizes a supremum of the risk function among any estimator. Namely, $\hat{\theta}_0$ is said to be minimax if

$$\sup_{\theta \in \mathcal{P}} R(\hat{\theta}_0, \theta) \leq \sup_{\theta \in \mathcal{P}} R(\hat{\theta}, \theta)$$

for any estimator $\hat{\theta}$. If an estimator $\hat{\theta}$ is better than a minimax estimator, then $\hat{\theta}$ is also minimax.

For a general explanation on decision-theoretic estimation, see, for example, Ferguson (1967) and Lehmann and Casella (1998). Clearly, admissibility and minimaxity strongly depend on loss functions, and there exists some criticism concerning criteria based on loss functions. Berger (1985) and Robert (2007) discussed some criticism on decision-theoretic estimation and the use of loss functions.

1.2 James-Stein's Shrinkage Estimator

Now, we look at the problem of estimating the mean vector $\boldsymbol{\theta}$ of p-variate normal distribution with the identity covariance matrix relative to the quadratic loss $L(\widehat{\boldsymbol{\theta}}, \boldsymbol{\theta}) = \|\widehat{\boldsymbol{\theta}} - \boldsymbol{\theta}\|^2$, where $\|\cdot\|$ denotes the Euclidean norm and $\widehat{\boldsymbol{\theta}}$ is an estimator of $\boldsymbol{\theta}$. A random vector drawn from the p-variate normal distribution is denoted by $\boldsymbol{X}$.

In estimation of the normal mean vector $\boldsymbol{\theta}$, the maximum likelihood estimator is $\widehat{\boldsymbol{\theta}}^{ML} = \boldsymbol{X}$, which is the uniformly minimum variance unbiased estimator. Also, $\widehat{\boldsymbol{\theta}}^{ML}$ is the best invariant estimator under the group of the affine transformations

$$\boldsymbol{X} \to \boldsymbol{A}\boldsymbol{X} + \boldsymbol{b}, \quad \boldsymbol{\theta} \to \boldsymbol{A}\boldsymbol{\theta} + \boldsymbol{b}, \tag{1.1}$$

where $\boldsymbol{A}$ is a $p \times p$ orthogonal matrix and $\boldsymbol{b}$ is a p-dimensional vector, and it is minimax with the constant risk p. From the above facts, $\widehat{\boldsymbol{\theta}}^{ML}$ has been recognized to be optimal for a long time. However, Stein (1956) showed that $\widehat{\boldsymbol{\theta}}^{ML}$ is inadmissible for three or more dimensional cases. Further James and Stein (1961) succeeded in providing an explicit estimator which dominates $\widehat{\boldsymbol{\theta}}^{ML}$. The dominating estimator is of the form

$$\widehat{\boldsymbol{\theta}}^{JS} = \left(1 - \frac{p-2}{\|\boldsymbol{X}\|^2}\right)\boldsymbol{X},$$

which is invariant under a subgroup of (1.1), $\boldsymbol{X} \to \boldsymbol{A}\boldsymbol{X}$ and $\boldsymbol{\theta} \to \boldsymbol{A}\boldsymbol{\theta}$ for a $p \times p$ orthogonal matrix $\boldsymbol{A}$. James and Stein's estimator $\widehat{\boldsymbol{\theta}}^{JS}$ is called a shrinkage estimator since it is shrinking $\widehat{\boldsymbol{\theta}}^{ML}$ toward the origin. James and Stein (1961) showed that the risk function of $\widehat{\boldsymbol{\theta}}^{JS}$ can be expressed as

$$R(\widehat{\boldsymbol{\theta}}^{JS}, \boldsymbol{\theta}) = p - (p-2)^2 E\left[(p-2+2K)^{-1}\right], \tag{1.2}$$

where K is a Poisson random variable with mean $\|\boldsymbol{\theta}\|^2/2$. The expectation in the r.h.s. of (1.2) is finite when $p \geq 3$, and then $R(\widehat{\boldsymbol{\theta}}^{JS}, \boldsymbol{\theta}) \leq R(\widehat{\boldsymbol{\theta}}^{ML}, \boldsymbol{\theta})$ for any $\boldsymbol{\theta}$, namely, $\widehat{\boldsymbol{\theta}}^{ML}$ is inadmissible relative to the quadratic loss L.

James and Stein's shrinkage estimator can be characterized by an empirical Bayes method as shown by Efron and Morris (1973). See Gruber (1998), who compared the shrinkage and the ML estimators for some linear models from the Bayesian and Frequentist points of view. A broad survey on shrinkage estimation is presented by Kubokawa (1998) and a modern Bayesian approach is explained extensively by Fourdrinier et al. (2018). For geometrical interpretation of the shrinkage estimator, see Brown and Zhao (2012).

1.3 Unbiased Risk Estimate and Stein's Identity

When $\boldsymbol{X}$ follows the p-variate normal distribution with mean $\boldsymbol{\theta}$ and the identity covariance matrix $\|\boldsymbol{X}\|^2$ is distributed as the noncentral chi-square distribution with p degrees of freedom and the noncentrality parameter $\|\boldsymbol{\theta}\|^2$. The p.d.f. of the noncentral chi-square distribution is written as a Poisson mixture and $E[\|\boldsymbol{X}\|^{-2}] = E[(p-2+2K)^{-1}]$, where K is the Poisson random variable defined in the previous section. The risk function of $\widehat{\boldsymbol{\theta}}^{JS}$ can be rewritten as $R(\widehat{\boldsymbol{\theta}}^{JS}, \boldsymbol{\theta}) = E[\widehat{R}^{JS}(\boldsymbol{X})]$, where

$$\widehat{R}^{JS}(\boldsymbol{x}) = p - \frac{(p-2)^2}{\|\boldsymbol{x}\|^2}.$$

Here $\widehat{R}^{JS}(\boldsymbol{x})$ is a function of p-dimensional vector $\boldsymbol{x}$ but independent of $\boldsymbol{\theta}$. Therefore it is called the unbiased risk estimate for $R(\widehat{\boldsymbol{\theta}}^{JS}, \boldsymbol{\theta})$. The unbiased risk estimate for $R(\widehat{\boldsymbol{\theta}}^{ML}, \boldsymbol{\theta})$ is given by $\widehat{R}^{ML}(\boldsymbol{x}) = p$, so that $\widehat{R}^{JS}(\boldsymbol{x}) \leq \widehat{R}^{ML}(\boldsymbol{x})$ for any $\boldsymbol{x}$ except when $\|\boldsymbol{x}\| = 0$.

The unbiased risk estimate provides simple methods of proving the inadmissibility of estimators and of finding better estimators. In fact, if there exist unbiased risk estimates $\widehat{R}_1(\boldsymbol{x})$ and $\widehat{R}_2(\boldsymbol{x})$ with respect to two estimators $\widehat{\boldsymbol{\theta}}_1$ and $\widehat{\boldsymbol{\theta}}_2$, respectively, such that $\widehat{R}_1(\boldsymbol{x}) \leq \widehat{R}_2(\boldsymbol{x})$ for any $\boldsymbol{x}$, then $R(\widehat{\boldsymbol{\theta}}_1, \boldsymbol{\theta}) \leq R(\widehat{\boldsymbol{\theta}}_2, \boldsymbol{\theta})$ uniformly for any $\boldsymbol{\theta}$.

In general, unbiased risk estimates are hard to derive. When we consider the class of estimators of the form $\widehat{\boldsymbol{\theta}}^G = \widehat{\boldsymbol{\theta}}^{ML} + \boldsymbol{G}$ with a vector-valued function $\boldsymbol{G}$ of $\boldsymbol{X}$, the risk function of $\widehat{\boldsymbol{\theta}}^G$ is expressed by

$$R(\widehat{\boldsymbol{\theta}}^G, \boldsymbol{\theta}) = R(\widehat{\boldsymbol{\theta}}^{ML}, \boldsymbol{\theta}) + E[\|\boldsymbol{G}\|^2 + 2(\boldsymbol{X} - \boldsymbol{\theta})^\top \boldsymbol{G}].$$

Therefore we need to evaluate $E[(\boldsymbol{X} - \boldsymbol{\theta})^\top \boldsymbol{G}]$ for deriving an unbiased risk estimate of $R(\widehat{\boldsymbol{\theta}}^G, \boldsymbol{\theta})$. To this end, Stein (1973, 1981) proved a useful integration by parts formula in terms of a normal distribution: Let x be a normal random variable with mean θ and variance one. Let g be an absolutely continuous function such that $E[(x - \theta)g(x)]$ and $E[g'(x)]$ are finite. Then the integration by parts formula is given by

$$E[(x - \theta)g(x)] = E[g'(x)], \tag{1.3}$$

which enables us to evaluate $E[(\boldsymbol{X} - \boldsymbol{\theta})^\top \boldsymbol{G}]$ given above.

The integration by parts formula (1.3) is named the Stein identity or the Stein lemma after Stein (1973, 1981). The Stein identity is nowadays a key tool for evaluating risk functions and for deriving unbiased risk estimates, and it has exerted an immeasurable influence on the development of shrinkage estimation.

References

J.O. Berger, *Statistical Decision Theory and Bayesian Analysis*, 2nd edn. (Springer, New York, 1985)

L.D. Brown, L.H. Zhao, A geometrical explanation of Stein shrinkage. Stat. Sci. **27**, 24–30 (2012)

B. Efron, C. Morris, Stein's estimation rule and its competitors—An empirical Bayes approach. J. Am. Stat. Assoc. **68**, 117–130 (1973)

T.S. Ferguson, *Mathematical Statistics: A Decision Theoretic Approach* (Academic Press, New York, 1967)

D. Fourdrinier, W.E. Strawderman, M.T. Wells, *Shrinkage Estimation* (Springer, New York, 2018)

M.H.J. Gruber, *Improving Efficiency by Shrinkage* (Marcel Dekker, New York, 1998)

W. James, C. Stein, Estimation with quadratic loss, in *proceedings of the Fourth Berkeley Symposium on Mathematical Statistics and Probability*, ed. by J. Neyman, vol. 1 (University of California Press, Berkeley, 1961), pp. 361–379

T. Kubokawa, The Stein phenomenon in simultaneous estimation: A review, in *Applied Statistical Science III*, ed. by S.E. Ahmed, M. Ahsanullah, B.K. Sinha (Nova Science Publishers, New York, 1998), pp. 143–173

E.L. Lehmann, G. Casella, *Theory of Point Estimation*, 2nd edn. (Springer, New York, 1998)

C. Robert, *The Bayesian Choice*, 2nd edn. (Springer, New York, 2007)

C. Stein, Inadmissibility of the usual estimator for the mean of a multivariate normal distribution, *Proceedings of the Third Berkeley Symposium on Mathematical Statistics and Probability*, ed. by J. Neyman, vol. 1 (University of California Press, Berkeley, 1956), pp. 197–206

C. Stein, Estimation of the mean of a multivariate normal distribution, Technical Reports No.48 (Department of Statistics, Stanford University, Stanford, 1973)

C. Stein, Estimation of the mean of a multivariate normal distribution. Ann. Stat. **9**, 1135–1151 (1981)

Chapter 2
Matrix Algebra

Matrix algebra is an important step in mathematical treatment of shrinkage estimation for matrix parameters, and in particular the Moore-Penrose inverse and some matrix decompositions are required for defining matricial shrinkage estimators. This chapter first explains the notation used in this book and subsequently lists helpful results in matrix algebra.

2.1 Notation

Let $\mathbb{R}^n$ be the n-dimensional real vector space and in particular denote $\mathbb{R} = \mathbb{R}^1$. Let $\mathbb{R}^{m\times n}$ be the set of all $m \times n$ matrices with real elements. Note that $\mathbb{R}^{m\times n} \neq \mathbb{R}^{mn}$ and $\mathbb{R}^{mn}$ is the (mn)-dimensional real vector space. If $\boldsymbol{A} \in \mathbb{R}^{m\times n}$ then $\boldsymbol{A}$ is of the form

$$\boldsymbol{A} = \begin{pmatrix} a_{11} & \cdots & a_{1n} \\ \vdots & & \vdots \\ a_{m1} & \cdots & a_{mn} \end{pmatrix},$$

where all the a_{ij}'s belong to $\mathbb{R}$ for $i = 1, \dots, m$ and $j = 1, \dots, n$. In some cases, $\boldsymbol{A}$ given above is written as $\boldsymbol{A} = (a_{ij})$, or $\boldsymbol{A} = (\boldsymbol{a}_1, \dots, \boldsymbol{a}_n)$ where for $j = 1, \dots, n$

$$\boldsymbol{a}_j = \begin{pmatrix} a_{1j} \\ \vdots \\ a_{mj} \end{pmatrix} \in \mathbb{R}^m.$$

Also, the (i, j)-th element of $\boldsymbol{A}$ is sometimes expressed as $a_{i,j}$ or $\{\boldsymbol{A}\}_{ij}$.

H. Tsukuma and T. Kubokawa, *Shrinkage Estimation for Mean and Covariance Matrices*, JSS Research Series in Statistics, https://doi.org/10.1007/978-981-15-1596-5_2

Let $\mathbf{0}_{m\times n}$ be the zero matrix of size $m \times n$. The diagonal matrix of size $n \times n$ is denoted by $\mathrm{diag}\,(d_1, \ldots, d_n)$, where $d_1, \ldots, d_n$ are diagonal elements from the upper left corner to the lower right one. Define the identity matrix of size $n \times n$ as $\boldsymbol{I}_n$, namely, $\boldsymbol{I}_n = \mathrm{diag}\,(1, \ldots, 1)$ consisting of n ones on the diagonal.

Let $\boldsymbol{A}^\top$ be the transpose of a matrix $\boldsymbol{A}$ and let $\mathrm{tr}\,\boldsymbol{A}$ and $|\boldsymbol{A}|$ be, respectively, the trace and the determinant of a square matrix $\boldsymbol{A}$. Also, let $\boldsymbol{A}^{-1}$ be the inverse of a nonsingular matrix $\boldsymbol{A}$. A matrix square root of a symmetric positive semi-definite matrix $\boldsymbol{A}$ is written as $\boldsymbol{A}^{1/2}$, where $\boldsymbol{A}^{1/2}$ is symmetric such that $\boldsymbol{A}^{1/2}\boldsymbol{A}^{1/2} = \boldsymbol{A}$. The inverse of $\boldsymbol{A}^{1/2}$ is expressed as $\boldsymbol{A}^{-1/2}$ if it exists.

We list the notation for special subsets in $\mathbb{R}^{m\times n}$ as follows:

$\mathbb{U}_n$: Set of all $n \times n$ nonsingular matrices;
$\mathbb{O}_n$: Set of all $n \times n$ orthogonal matrices;
$\mathbb{V}_{m,n}$: Set of all $m \times n$ matrices $\boldsymbol{A}$ such that $\boldsymbol{A}^\top\boldsymbol{A} = \boldsymbol{I}_n$ for $m \geq n$;
$\mathbb{D}_n$: Set of all $n \times n$ diagonal matrices;
$\mathbb{D}_n^{(\geq)}$: Set of all $n \times n$ diagonal matrices $\mathrm{diag}\,(d_1, \ldots, d_n)$ such that $d_1 \geq \cdots \geq d_n$;
$\mathbb{D}_n^{(\geq 0)}$: Set of all $n \times n$ diagonal matrices $\mathrm{diag}\,(d_1, \ldots, d_n)$ such that $d_1 \geq \cdots \geq d_n \geq 0$;
$\mathbb{L}_n^{(+)}$: Set of all $n \times n$ lower triangular matrices with positive diagonal elements;
$\mathbb{L}_n^{(1)}$: Set of all $n \times n$ lower triangular matrices with ones on the diagonal;
$\mathbb{L}_{m,n}^{(+)}$: Set of all $m \times n$ matrices of the form

$$\boldsymbol{A} = \begin{pmatrix} \boldsymbol{A}_1 \\ \boldsymbol{A}_2 \end{pmatrix},$$

where $m \geq n$, $\boldsymbol{A}_1 \in \mathbb{L}_n^{(+)}$ and $\boldsymbol{A}_2 \in \mathbb{R}^{(m-n)\times n}$;
$\mathbb{L}_{m,n}^{(1)}$: Set of all $m \times n$ matrices $\boldsymbol{A} = (a_{ij}) \in \mathbb{L}_{m,n}^{(+)}$ such that $a_{ii} = 1$ for $i = 1, \ldots, n$;
$\mathbb{S}_n$: Set of all $n \times n$ symmetric matrices;
$\mathbb{S}_n^{(+)}$: Set of all $n \times n$ symmetric positive definite matrices;
$\mathbb{S}_{n,r}^{(+)}$: Set of all $n \times n$ symmetric positive semi-definite matrices with rank r.

Note that $\mathbb{O}_n = \mathbb{V}_{n,n}$, $\mathbb{L}_n^{(+)} = \mathbb{L}_{n,n}^{(+)}$, $\mathbb{L}_n^{(1)} = \mathbb{L}_{n,n}^{(1)}$ and $\mathbb{S}_n^{(+)} = \mathbb{S}_{n,n}^{(+)}$. Set $\mathbb{V}_{m,n}$ is referred to as the Stiefel manifold. Also, it is important to note that $\mathbb{O}_n$ and $\mathbb{L}_n^{(+)}$ are groups, called respectively the orthogonal and the lower triangular groups, with respect to the group action by usual matrix multiplication.

Matrix inequality is defined in the Löwner sense. Namely, for $\boldsymbol{A}_1, \boldsymbol{A}_2 \in \mathbb{S}_n$, the matrix inequality $\boldsymbol{A}_1 \preceq \boldsymbol{A}_2$ (or $\boldsymbol{A}_1 \succeq \boldsymbol{A}_2$) means that $\boldsymbol{A}_2 - \boldsymbol{A}_1$ (or $\boldsymbol{A}_1 - \boldsymbol{A}_2$) is symmetric positive semi-definite.

For definition, concepts and applications in terms of matrix algebra, see, for example, Rao (1973), Golub and Van Loan (1996) and Harville (1997).

2.2 Nonsingular Matrix and the Moore-Penrose Inverse

A matrix $\boldsymbol{A} \in \mathbb{R}^{n\times n}$ is said to be invertible if there exists a matrix $\boldsymbol{B} \in \mathbb{R}^{n\times n}$ such that $\boldsymbol{AB} = \boldsymbol{BA} = \boldsymbol{I}_n$. Such a matrix $\boldsymbol{B}$ is uniquely defined from $\boldsymbol{A}$ and is denoted by $\boldsymbol{A}^{-1}$, called the inverse of $\boldsymbol{A}$. A matrix $\boldsymbol{A}$ is invertible if and only if $\boldsymbol{A}$ belongs to $\mathbb{U}_n$, namely, $|\boldsymbol{A}| \neq 0$, and thus an invertible matrix is also called a nonsingular matrix. Here we give an important result on the inverse of a partitioned matrix.

Lemma 2.1 *Partition* $\boldsymbol{A} \in \mathbb{R}^{n\times n}$ *as*

$$\boldsymbol{A} = \begin{pmatrix} \boldsymbol{A}_{11} & \boldsymbol{A}_{12} \\ \boldsymbol{A}_{21} & \boldsymbol{A}_{22} \end{pmatrix},$$

where $\boldsymbol{A}_{11}$, $\boldsymbol{A}_{12}$, $\boldsymbol{A}_{21}$ *and* $\boldsymbol{A}_{22}$ *are matrix subblocks of any size. If* $\boldsymbol{A}_{11}$ *and* $\boldsymbol{A}_{22\cdot 1} = \boldsymbol{A}_{22} - \boldsymbol{A}_{21}\boldsymbol{A}_{11}^{-1}\boldsymbol{A}_{12}$ *are squared and nonsingular then* $\boldsymbol{A}$ *is nonsingular and*

$$\boldsymbol{A}^{-1} = \begin{pmatrix} \boldsymbol{A}_{11}^{-1} + \boldsymbol{A}_{11}^{-1}\boldsymbol{A}_{12}\boldsymbol{A}_{22\cdot 1}^{-1}\boldsymbol{A}_{21}\boldsymbol{A}_{11}^{-1} & -\boldsymbol{A}_{11}^{-1}\boldsymbol{A}_{12}\boldsymbol{A}_{22\cdot 1}^{-1} \\ -\boldsymbol{A}_{22\cdot 1}^{-1}\boldsymbol{A}_{21}\boldsymbol{A}_{11}^{-1} & \boldsymbol{A}_{22\cdot 1}^{-1} \end{pmatrix}.$$

In addition, if $\boldsymbol{A}_{22}$ *and* $\boldsymbol{A}_{11\cdot 2} = \boldsymbol{A}_{11} - \boldsymbol{A}_{12}\boldsymbol{A}_{22}^{-1}\boldsymbol{A}_{21}$ *are also nonsingular then*

$$\boldsymbol{A}_{11}^{-1} + \boldsymbol{A}_{11}^{-1}\boldsymbol{A}_{12}\boldsymbol{A}_{22\cdot 1}^{-1}\boldsymbol{A}_{21}\boldsymbol{A}_{11}^{-1} = \boldsymbol{A}_{11\cdot 2}^{-1}.$$

In particular, if $\boldsymbol{A} \in \mathbb{S}_n^{(+)}$ *then* $\boldsymbol{A}_{11}$, $\boldsymbol{A}_{22}$, $\boldsymbol{A}_{11\cdot 2}$ *and* $\boldsymbol{A}_{22\cdot 1}$ *are nonsingular.*

If a matrix $\boldsymbol{A}$ is partitioned as in Lemma 2.1 and $\boldsymbol{A}_{11} \in \mathbb{U}_m$ with $m < n$, then $\boldsymbol{A}$ can be expressed as

$$\boldsymbol{A} = \begin{pmatrix} \boldsymbol{I}_m & \boldsymbol{0}_{m\times(n-m)} \\ \boldsymbol{A}_{21}\boldsymbol{A}_{11}^{-1} & \boldsymbol{I}_{n-m} \end{pmatrix} \begin{pmatrix} \boldsymbol{A}_{11} & \boldsymbol{0}_{m\times(n-m)} \\ \boldsymbol{0}_{(n-m)\times m} & \boldsymbol{A}_{22\cdot 1} \end{pmatrix} \begin{pmatrix} \boldsymbol{I}_m & \boldsymbol{A}_{11}^{-1}\boldsymbol{A}_{12} \\ \boldsymbol{0}_{(n-m)\times m} & \boldsymbol{I}_{n-m} \end{pmatrix}. \quad (2.1)$$

Therefore Lemma 2.1 can easily be verified by (2.1).

Next, we describe some basic and useful properties of the Moore-Penrose inverse, which will be needed for a unified treatment of high- and low-dimensional shrinkage estimators. The Moore-Penrose inverse is an extension of invertibility to a singular square matrix and to a rectangular matrix, and further it is a special case of generalized inverse. Here, for a matrix $\boldsymbol{A} \in \mathbb{R}^{m\times n}$, a matrix $\boldsymbol{A}^-$ $(\in \mathbb{R}^{n\times m})$ is said to be a generalized inverse of $\boldsymbol{A}$ if $\boldsymbol{A}^-$ satisfies $\boldsymbol{AA}^-\boldsymbol{A} = \boldsymbol{A}$. The generalized inverse is not unique, while the Moore-Penrose inverse is unique.

Definition 2.1 For a matrix $\boldsymbol{A}$ $(\in \mathbb{R}^{m\times n})$, a matrix $\boldsymbol{A}^+$ $(\in \mathbb{R}^{n\times m})$ is called the Moore-Penrose inverse of $\boldsymbol{A}$ if $\boldsymbol{A}^+$ satisfies

(i) $\boldsymbol{AA}^+\boldsymbol{A} = \boldsymbol{A}$,
(ii) $\boldsymbol{A}^+\boldsymbol{AA}^+ = \boldsymbol{A}^+$,

(iii) $(\boldsymbol{A}\boldsymbol{A}^{+})^{\top} = \boldsymbol{A}\boldsymbol{A}^{+}$,
(iv) $(\boldsymbol{A}^{+}\boldsymbol{A})^{\top} = \boldsymbol{A}^{+}\boldsymbol{A}$.

Lemma 2.2 *For any matrix $\boldsymbol{A}$, $\boldsymbol{A}^{+}$ always exists and it is unique.*

Lemma 2.3 *For $m \geq n$, let $\boldsymbol{A} \in \mathbb{R}^{m\times n}$ be of full column rank. Then we have*

(i) $\boldsymbol{A}^{+} = (\boldsymbol{A}^{\top}\boldsymbol{A})^{-1}\boldsymbol{A}^{\top} \in \mathbb{R}^{n\times m}$, *and in particular* $\boldsymbol{A}^{+} = \boldsymbol{A}^{\top}$ *if* $\boldsymbol{A} \in \mathbb{V}_{m,n}$,
(ii) $(\boldsymbol{A}^{\top})^{+} = \boldsymbol{A}(\boldsymbol{A}^{\top}\boldsymbol{A})^{-1}$, *and thus* $(\boldsymbol{A}^{\top})^{+} = (\boldsymbol{A}^{+})^{\top}$,
(iii) $\boldsymbol{A}^{+}\boldsymbol{A} = \boldsymbol{I}_n$,
(iv) $(\boldsymbol{A}\boldsymbol{B}\boldsymbol{A}^{\top})^{+} = (\boldsymbol{A}^{\top})^{+}\boldsymbol{B}^{-1}\boldsymbol{A}^{+}$ *for any* $\boldsymbol{B} \in \mathbb{U}_n$.

Parts (i) and (ii) of Lemma 2.3 can easily be verified by Definition 2.1 and Lemma 2.2. Part (iii) can be obtained from (i). Part (iv) follows from Definition 2.1 and Lemma 2.2 with (ii) and (iii).

Using (i) of Lemma 2.3, we can see that if $\boldsymbol{A} \in \mathbb{U}_n$ then $\boldsymbol{A}^{+} = (\boldsymbol{A}^{\top}\boldsymbol{A})^{-1}\boldsymbol{A}^{\top} = \boldsymbol{A}^{-1}(\boldsymbol{A}^{\top})^{-1}\boldsymbol{A}^{\top} = \boldsymbol{A}^{-1}$. This implies that if $\boldsymbol{A} \in \mathbb{U}_n$ and it is symmetric then $\boldsymbol{A}^{+}$ is symmetric as well. For more general results on the Moore-Penrose inverse, see Harville (1997) and Magnus and Neudecker (1999).

2.3 Kronecker Product and Vec Operator

The notion of the Kronecker product and the vec operator is very important to discuss a clear theorization in terms of matrix-variate distributions. Here, we provide their definition and list some useful results without proofs. For the proofs and more details, see Harville (1997) and Muirhead (1982).

Definition 2.2 The Kronecker product of two matrices $\boldsymbol{A} = (a_{ij}) \in \mathbb{R}^{m\times n}$ and $\boldsymbol{B} \in \mathbb{R}^{p\times q}$ is denoted by $\boldsymbol{A} \otimes \boldsymbol{B}$, which is a block matrix of the form

$$\boldsymbol{A} \otimes \boldsymbol{B} = \begin{pmatrix} a_{11}\boldsymbol{B} & a_{12}\boldsymbol{B} & \cdots & a_{1n}\boldsymbol{B} \\ a_{21}\boldsymbol{B} & a_{22}\boldsymbol{B} & \cdots & a_{2n}\boldsymbol{B} \\ \vdots & \vdots & \ddots & \vdots \\ a_{m1}\boldsymbol{B} & a_{m2}\boldsymbol{B} & \cdots & a_{mn}\boldsymbol{B} \end{pmatrix} \in \mathbb{R}^{mp\times nq}.$$

Lemma 2.4 *Some results on the Kronecker product are given as follows:*

(i) $(\boldsymbol{A} \otimes \boldsymbol{B})(\boldsymbol{C} \otimes \boldsymbol{D}) = \boldsymbol{A}\boldsymbol{C} \otimes \boldsymbol{B}\boldsymbol{D}$ *for* $\boldsymbol{A} \in \mathbb{R}^{m\times n}$, $\boldsymbol{B} \in \mathbb{R}^{p\times q}$, $\boldsymbol{C} \in \mathbb{R}^{n\times r}$ *and* $\boldsymbol{D} \in \mathbb{R}^{q\times s}$,
(ii) $(\boldsymbol{A} \otimes \boldsymbol{B})^{\top} = \boldsymbol{A}^{\top} \otimes \boldsymbol{B}^{\top}$,
(iii) $|\boldsymbol{A} \otimes \boldsymbol{B}| = |\boldsymbol{A}|^{n}|\boldsymbol{B}|^{m}$ *for* $\boldsymbol{A} \in \mathbb{R}^{m\times m}$ *and* $\boldsymbol{B} \in \mathbb{R}^{n\times n}$,
(iv) $(\boldsymbol{A} \otimes \boldsymbol{B})^{-1} = \boldsymbol{A}^{-1} \otimes \boldsymbol{B}^{-1}$ *for nonsingular matrices* $\boldsymbol{A}$ *and* $\boldsymbol{B}$.

Definition 2.3 Let $\boldsymbol{A} = (\boldsymbol{a}_1, \ldots, \boldsymbol{a}_n) \in \mathbb{R}^{m\times n}$, where the $\boldsymbol{a}_i$'s lie in $\mathbb{R}^m$. The vec operation on $\boldsymbol{A}$ is expressed by $\mathrm{vec}(\boldsymbol{A})$, which is of the form

$$\mathrm{vec}(\boldsymbol{A}) = \begin{pmatrix} \boldsymbol{a}_1 \\ \vdots \\ \boldsymbol{a}_n \end{pmatrix} \in \mathbb{R}^{mn}.$$

Lemma 2.5 *Some results on the vec operation are given as follows:*

(i) If $\boldsymbol{A} \in \mathbb{R}^{m\times n}$, $\boldsymbol{X} \in \mathbb{R}^{n\times p}$ and $\boldsymbol{B} \in \mathbb{R}^{p\times q}$ then

$$\mathrm{vec}(\boldsymbol{AXB}) = (\boldsymbol{B}^\top \otimes \boldsymbol{A})\mathrm{vec}(\boldsymbol{X}).$$

(ii) If $\boldsymbol{X} \in \mathbb{R}^{m\times n}$, $\boldsymbol{A} \in \mathbb{R}^{m\times m}$ and $\boldsymbol{B} \in \mathbb{R}^{n\times n}$ then

$$\mathrm{tr}\,\boldsymbol{AXBX}^\top = \mathrm{vec}(\boldsymbol{X})^\top(\boldsymbol{B}^\top \otimes \boldsymbol{A})\mathrm{vec}(\boldsymbol{X}) = \mathrm{vec}(\boldsymbol{X})^\top(\boldsymbol{B} \otimes \boldsymbol{A}^\top)\mathrm{vec}(\boldsymbol{X}).$$

2.4 Matrix Decompositions

A matrix decomposition, or a matrix factorization, is to express a matrix as a product of some matrices. The matrix decomposition appears in various scenes of statistical analysis. In shrinkage estimation, it is often used for finding better estimators. This section provides some important matrix decompositions without proofs. For the proofs and properties of matrix decompositions, see Golub and Van Loan (1996) and Harville (1997).

Lemma 2.6 (QR decomposition) *Let $\boldsymbol{A} \in \mathbb{R}^{m\times n}$ be of full column rank. Then there exist unique $\boldsymbol{R} \in \mathbb{L}_n^{(+)}$ and $\boldsymbol{Q} \in \mathbb{V}_{m,n}$ such that $\boldsymbol{A} = \boldsymbol{QR}^\top$.*

The QR decomposition $\boldsymbol{A} = \boldsymbol{QR}^\top$ yields $\boldsymbol{A}^\top = \boldsymbol{RQ}^\top$, implying that for $\boldsymbol{A} \in \mathbb{R}^{m\times n}$ of full row rank there exist unique $\boldsymbol{L} \in \mathbb{L}_m^{(+)}$ and $\boldsymbol{Q} \in \mathbb{V}_{n,m}$ such that $\boldsymbol{A} = \boldsymbol{LQ}^\top$. The decomposition $\boldsymbol{A} = \boldsymbol{LQ}^\top$ is called the LQ decomposition.

Lemma 2.7 (Cholesky decomposition) *For any $\boldsymbol{A} \in \mathbb{S}_n^{(+)}$, there exists a unique $\boldsymbol{L} \in \mathbb{L}_n^{(+)}$ such that $\boldsymbol{A} = \boldsymbol{LL}^\top$.*

If $\boldsymbol{A} \in \mathbb{S}_n^{(+)}$ then $\boldsymbol{A}$ can also be decomposed as $\boldsymbol{A} = \boldsymbol{LDL}^\top$, where $\boldsymbol{L} \in \mathbb{L}_n^{(1)}$, $\boldsymbol{D} \in \mathbb{D}_n$ with positive diagonals, and $\boldsymbol{L}$ and $\boldsymbol{D}$ are unique. This is known as the LDL$^\top$ decomposition.

When $\boldsymbol{A} \in \mathbb{R}^{n\times n}$ can be decomposed as $\boldsymbol{A} = \boldsymbol{LU}$, where $\boldsymbol{L}$ and $\boldsymbol{U}$ are, respectively, lower and upper triangular matrices, the decomposition is called the LU decomposition of $\boldsymbol{A}$.

Lemma 2.8 (Eigenvalue decomposition) *For any $\boldsymbol{A} \in \mathbb{R}^{n\times n}$, there exists $\boldsymbol{P} \in \mathbb{U}_n$ such that $\boldsymbol{A} = \boldsymbol{PDP}^{-1}$, where $\boldsymbol{D} \in \mathbb{D}_n^{(\geq)}$. In particular, if $\boldsymbol{A} \in \mathbb{S}_{n,r}^{(+)}$ then there exist $\boldsymbol{D} \in \mathbb{D}_r^{(\geq 0)}$ and $\boldsymbol{P} \in \mathbb{V}_{n,r}$ such that $\boldsymbol{A} = \boldsymbol{PDP}^\top$.*

The eigenvalue decomposition is also named spectral decomposition. The diagonal elements of $\boldsymbol{D}$ in Lemma 2.8 are called the eigenvalues of $\boldsymbol{A}$ and the i-th column of $\boldsymbol{P}$ is called the eigenvector corresponding to the i-th diagonal element of $\boldsymbol{D}$. The eigenvalue and eigenvector are also referred to as the characteristic root and characteristic vector, respectively. The eigenvalues of $\boldsymbol{A}$ are arranged in descending order on the diagonal of $\boldsymbol{D}$, implying that $\boldsymbol{D}$ is uniquely determined. When $\boldsymbol{A}$ is a member of $\mathbb{S}_{n,r}^{(+)}$, $\boldsymbol{D}$ is unique and $\boldsymbol{P}$ is also unique up to sign changes of columns of $\boldsymbol{P}$.

Lemma 2.9 (Singular value decomposition) *For any $\boldsymbol{A} \in \mathbb{R}^{m\times n}$ with rank r, there exist $\boldsymbol{D} \in \mathbb{D}_r^{(\geq 0)}$, $\boldsymbol{U} \in \mathbb{V}_{m,r}$ and $\boldsymbol{V} \in \mathbb{V}_{n,r}$ such that $\boldsymbol{A} = \boldsymbol{U}\boldsymbol{D}\boldsymbol{V}^\top$.*

The diagonal elements of $\boldsymbol{D}$ in Lemma 2.9 are called the singular values of $\boldsymbol{A}$. The singular value decomposition $\boldsymbol{A} = \boldsymbol{U}\boldsymbol{D}\boldsymbol{V}^\top$ is unique up to sign changes of columns of $\boldsymbol{V}$.

Here we introduce the wedge and descending wedge symbols, $\wedge$ and $\vee$, implying that, for numbers a and b,

$$a \wedge b = \min(a, b), \qquad a \vee b = \max(a, b).$$

Also for numbers a, b and c, $a \wedge b \wedge c = \min(a, b, c)$. The following identities hold:

$$a \vee b - (a \wedge b) = |a - b| = a + b - 2(a \wedge b) = 2(a \vee b) - a - b.$$

If $\boldsymbol{A} \in \mathbb{R}^{m\times n}$ is of full rank, then its rank is $m \wedge n$ and the singular value decomposition of $\boldsymbol{A}$ can be expressed by $\boldsymbol{A} = \boldsymbol{U}\boldsymbol{D}\boldsymbol{V}^\top$, where $\boldsymbol{D} \in \mathbb{D}_{m\wedge n}^{(\geq 0)}$, $\boldsymbol{U} \in \mathbb{V}_{m,m\wedge n}$ and $\boldsymbol{V} \in \mathbb{V}_{n,m\wedge n}$.

References

G.H. Golub, C.F. Van Loan, *Matrix Computations*, 3rd edn. (The Johns Hopkins University Press, Baltimore, 1996)

D.A. Harville, *Matrix Algebra From a Statistician's Perspective* (Springer, New York, 1997)

J.R. Magnus, H. Neudecker, *Matrix Differential Calculus with Applications in Statistics and Econometrics*, 2nd edn. (Wiley, New York, 1999)

R.J. Muirhead, *Aspects of Multivariate Statistical Theory* (Wiley, New York, 1982)

C.R. Rao, *Linear Statistical Inference and its Applications*, 2nd edn. (Wiley, New York, 1973)

Chapter 3
Matrix-Variate Distributions

This chapter provides the definition and some useful properties of a matrix-variate normal distribution, nonsingular and singular Wishart distributions, and other related distributions. The matrix-variate distributions considered here are based on the multivariate (vector-valued) normal distribution, and so we begin by briefly introducing the multivariate normal distribution and some Jacobians for matrix transformations used to obtain probability density functions of the matrix-variate distributions.

3.1 Preliminaries

3.1.1 The Multivariate Normal Distribution

A p-dimensional random vector follows a multivariate (vector-valued) normal distribution if the probability density function (p.d.f.) is given by

$$\frac{1}{(2\pi)^{p/2}|\boldsymbol{\Sigma}|^{1/2}} \exp\Big(-\frac{1}{2}(\boldsymbol{x}-\boldsymbol{\mu})^\top \boldsymbol{\Sigma}^{-1}(\boldsymbol{x}-\boldsymbol{\mu})\Big), \quad \boldsymbol{x} \in \mathbb{R}^p,$$

where $\boldsymbol{\mu}$ ($\in \mathbb{R}^p$) and $\boldsymbol{\Sigma}$ ($\in \mathbb{S}_p^{(+)}$) are parameters. Such a multivariate (p-variate) normal distribution is denoted by $\mathcal{N}_p(\boldsymbol{\mu}, \boldsymbol{\Sigma})$. The multivariate normal distribution has the following properties.

Lemma 3.1 *Let* $\boldsymbol{x} = (x_1, \dots, x_p)^\top \sim \mathcal{N}_p(\boldsymbol{\mu}, \boldsymbol{\Sigma})$ *with* $\boldsymbol{\mu} = (\mu_1, \dots, \mu_p)^\top \in \mathbb{R}^p$ *and* $\boldsymbol{\Sigma} = (\sigma_{ij}) \in \mathbb{S}_p^{(+)}$. *Then*

(i) $E[x_i] = \mu_i$ *and* $E[x_i x_j] = \mu_i\mu_j + \sigma_{ij}$ *for all* $i, j \in \{1, \dots, p\}$. *In other words,*

$$E[\boldsymbol{x}] = (E[x_1], \dots, E[x_p])^\top = \boldsymbol{\mu},$$
$$E[(\boldsymbol{x}-\boldsymbol{\mu})(\boldsymbol{x}-\boldsymbol{\mu})^\top] = \big(E[(x_i-\mu_i)(x_j-\mu_j)]\big) = \boldsymbol{\Sigma}.$$

H. Tsukuma and T. Kubokawa, *Shrinkage Estimation for Mean and Covariance Matrices*, JSS Research Series in Statistics, https://doi.org/10.1007/978-981-15-1596-5_3

(ii) *For a full row rank constant matrix* $\boldsymbol{A} \in \mathbb{R}^{q \times p}$ *and a constant vector* $\boldsymbol{b} \in \mathbb{R}^q$, $\boldsymbol{A}\boldsymbol{x} + \boldsymbol{b} \sim \mathcal{N}_q(\boldsymbol{A}\boldsymbol{\mu} + \boldsymbol{b}, \boldsymbol{A}\boldsymbol{\Sigma}\boldsymbol{A}^\top)$.

(iii) *If* $\boldsymbol{x}$, $\boldsymbol{\mu}$ *and* $\boldsymbol{\Sigma}$ *are partitioned, respectively, as*

$$\boldsymbol{x} = \begin{pmatrix} \boldsymbol{x}_1 \\ \boldsymbol{x}_2 \end{pmatrix}, \quad \boldsymbol{\mu} = \begin{pmatrix} \boldsymbol{\mu}_1 \\ \boldsymbol{\mu}_2 \end{pmatrix}, \quad \boldsymbol{\Sigma} = \begin{pmatrix} \boldsymbol{\Sigma}_{11} & \boldsymbol{\Sigma}_{21}^\top \\ \boldsymbol{\Sigma}_{21} & \boldsymbol{\Sigma}_{22} \end{pmatrix},$$

where $\boldsymbol{x}_1 \in \mathbb{R}^q$, $\boldsymbol{\mu}_1 \in \mathbb{R}^q$ *and* $\boldsymbol{\Sigma}_{11} \in \mathbb{S}_q^{(+)}$, *then*

$$\begin{aligned} \boldsymbol{x}_1 &\sim \mathcal{N}_q(\boldsymbol{\mu}_1, \boldsymbol{\Sigma}_{11}), \\ \boldsymbol{x}_2 | \boldsymbol{x}_1 &\sim \mathcal{N}_{p-q}(\boldsymbol{\mu}_2 + \boldsymbol{\Sigma}_{21}\boldsymbol{\Sigma}_{11}^{-1}(\boldsymbol{x}_1 - \boldsymbol{\mu}_1), \boldsymbol{\Sigma}_{22} - \boldsymbol{\Sigma}_{21}\boldsymbol{\Sigma}_{11}^{-1}\boldsymbol{\Sigma}_{21}^\top). \end{aligned}$$

Further, $\boldsymbol{x}_1$ *and* $\boldsymbol{x}_2$ *are independent if and only if* $\boldsymbol{\Sigma}_{21} = \boldsymbol{0}_{(p-q)\times q}$.

From (i) of Lemma 3.1, $\mathcal{N}_p(\boldsymbol{\mu}, \boldsymbol{\Sigma})$ is usually called the p-variate normal distribution with mean $\boldsymbol{\mu}$ and covariance $\boldsymbol{\Sigma}$. For theoretical properties other than Lemma 3.1, see Muirhead (1982) and Srivastava and Khatri (1979).

3.1.2 Jacobians of Matrix Transformations

Let $\boldsymbol{X}$ be a matrix such that it has k functionally independent variables x_i's and let $\boldsymbol{Y} = F(\boldsymbol{X})$ be a matrix transformation, where $\boldsymbol{Y}$ is a matrix having k functionally independent variables y_i's. The Jacobian of the transformation is given by $J(\boldsymbol{X} \to \boldsymbol{Y}) = |\boldsymbol{J}|$, where $\boldsymbol{J} = (\partial x_i / \partial y_j)$ is the $k \times k$ Jacobian matrix. Let $(\mathrm{d}\boldsymbol{X}) = \bigwedge_{i=1}^k \mathrm{d}x_i$ and $(\mathrm{d}\boldsymbol{Y}) = \bigwedge_{i=1}^k \mathrm{d}y_i$, where $\bigwedge$ denotes the exterior product. Then $(\mathrm{d}\boldsymbol{X}) = J(\boldsymbol{X} \to \boldsymbol{Y})(\mathrm{d}\boldsymbol{Y})$.

This section provides some specific Jacobians of matrix transformations. When considering a matrix transformation, we need to take attention to the number of functionally independent variables. For example, $\boldsymbol{S} = (s_{ij}) \in \mathbb{S}_n$ has $\{n(n+1)/2\}$ distinct elements, and the exterior product of distinct elements of the differential $\mathrm{d}\boldsymbol{S} = (\mathrm{d}s_{ij}) \in \mathbb{S}_n$ is $(\mathrm{d}\boldsymbol{S}) = \bigwedge_{i=1}^n \bigwedge_{j=1}^i \mathrm{d}s_{ij}$. See Muirhead (1982) and Mathai (1997) for more details of Jacobians and exterior products. Hereafter we ignore the signs of exterior differential forms and define only positive integrals.

Lemma 3.2 *Let* $\boldsymbol{X} = (x_{ij}) \in \mathbb{R}^{m \times n}$ *and* $\boldsymbol{Y} = (y_{ij}) \in \mathbb{R}^{m \times n}$. *If* $\boldsymbol{X} = \boldsymbol{A}\boldsymbol{Y}\boldsymbol{B} + \boldsymbol{C}$ *with* $\boldsymbol{A} \in \mathbb{U}_m$, $\boldsymbol{B} \in \mathbb{U}_n$ *and* $\boldsymbol{C} \in \mathbb{R}^{m \times n}$, *then* $(\mathrm{d}\boldsymbol{X}) = |\boldsymbol{A}|^n |\boldsymbol{B}|^m (\mathrm{d}\boldsymbol{Y})$, *where* $(\mathrm{d}\boldsymbol{X}) = \bigwedge_{i=1}^m \bigwedge_{j=1}^n \mathrm{d}x_{ij}$ *and* $(\mathrm{d}\boldsymbol{Y}) = \bigwedge_{i=1}^m \bigwedge_{j=1}^n \mathrm{d}y_{ij}$.

Proof See Muirhead (1982) and Mathai (1997). □

Lemma 3.3 *Let* $\boldsymbol{X} \in \mathbb{R}^{p \times n}$ *with full row rank. Denote by* $\boldsymbol{X} = \boldsymbol{T}\boldsymbol{Q}^\top$ *the LQ decomposition of* $\boldsymbol{X}$, *where* $\boldsymbol{T} = (t_{ij}) \in \mathbb{L}_p^{(+)}$ *and* $\boldsymbol{Q} \in \mathbb{V}_{n,p}$. *Then*

$$(\mathrm{d}\boldsymbol{X}) = \left(\prod_{i=1}^{p} t_{ii}^{n-i}\right)(\mathrm{d}\boldsymbol{T})(\boldsymbol{Q}^\top \mathrm{d}\boldsymbol{Q}),$$

where $(\mathrm{d}\boldsymbol{T}) = \bigwedge_{i=1}^{p} \bigwedge_{j=1}^{i} \mathrm{d}t_{ij}$ *and* $(\boldsymbol{Q}^\top \mathrm{d}\boldsymbol{Q})$ *is an unnormalized probability measure on* $\mathbb{V}_{n,p}$.

Proof See Muirhead (1982, Theorem 2.1.13). □

Muirhead (1982, p. 69) pointed out that the measure $(\boldsymbol{Q}^\top \mathrm{d}\boldsymbol{Q})$ on $\mathbb{V}_{n,p}$ is invariant under the orthogonal transformations $\boldsymbol{Q} \to \boldsymbol{A}\boldsymbol{Q}$ for $\boldsymbol{A} \in \mathbb{O}_n$ and $\boldsymbol{Q} \to \boldsymbol{Q}\boldsymbol{B}$ for $\boldsymbol{B} \in \mathbb{O}_p$. Also,

$$\int_{\mathbb{V}_{n,p}} (\boldsymbol{Q}^\top \mathrm{d}\boldsymbol{Q}) = \frac{2^p \pi^{np/2}}{\Gamma_p(n/2)}, \tag{3.1}$$

which is given in Muirhead (1982, Theorem 2.1.15), where $\Gamma_p(n/2)$ is the multivariate gamma function (see Definition 3.1 given below).

Lemma 3.4 *Let* $\boldsymbol{S} \in \mathbb{S}_p^{(+)}$ *and let* $\boldsymbol{S} = \boldsymbol{T}\boldsymbol{T}^\top$ *be the Cholesky decomposition of* $\boldsymbol{S}$, *where* $\boldsymbol{T} = (t_{ij}) \in \mathbb{L}_p^{(+)}$. *Then* $(\mathrm{d}\boldsymbol{S}) = 2^p(\prod_{i=1}^{p} t_{ii}^{p+1-i})(\mathrm{d}\boldsymbol{T})$.

Proof See Muirhead (1982, Theorem 2.1.9). □

Lemma 3.5 *Let* $\boldsymbol{S} \in \mathbb{S}_{p,r}^{(+)}$. *Denote by* $\boldsymbol{S} = \boldsymbol{H}\boldsymbol{L}\boldsymbol{H}^\top$ *the eigenvalue decomposition of* $\boldsymbol{S}$, *where* $\boldsymbol{L} = \mathrm{diag}(\ell_1, \ldots, \ell_r) \in \mathbb{D}_r^{(\geq 0)}$ *and* $\boldsymbol{H} \in \mathbb{V}_{p,r}$. *Then*

$$(\mathrm{d}\boldsymbol{S}) = \frac{1}{2^r}\left(\prod_{i=1}^{r} \ell_i^{p-r}\right)\left(\prod_{1 \leq i < j \leq r} (\ell_i - \ell_j)\right)(\mathrm{d}\boldsymbol{L})(\boldsymbol{H}^\top \mathrm{d}\boldsymbol{H}),$$

where $(\mathrm{d}\boldsymbol{L}) = \bigwedge_{i=1}^{r} \mathrm{d}\ell_i$.

Proof See Uhlig (1994, Theorem 2). □

Lemma 3.6 *Let* $\boldsymbol{X} \in \mathbb{R}^{p \times n}$ *with rank* r. *Denote by* $\boldsymbol{X} = \boldsymbol{U}\boldsymbol{D}\boldsymbol{V}^\top$ *the singular value decomposition of* $\boldsymbol{X}$, *where* $\boldsymbol{D} = \mathrm{diag}(d_1, \ldots, d_r) \in \mathbb{D}_r^{(\geq 0)}$, $\boldsymbol{U} \in \mathbb{V}_{p,r}$ *and* $\boldsymbol{V} \in \mathbb{V}_{n,r}$. *Then*

$$(\mathrm{d}\boldsymbol{X}) = \frac{1}{2^r}\left(\prod_{i=1}^{r} d_i^{p+n-2r}\right)\left(\prod_{1 \leq i < j \leq r} (d_i^2 - d_j^2)\right)(\boldsymbol{U}^\top \mathrm{d}\boldsymbol{U})(\mathrm{d}\boldsymbol{D})(\boldsymbol{V}^\top \mathrm{d}\boldsymbol{V}).$$

Proof See Díaz-García et al. (1997, Theorem 3.1). □

3.1.3 The Multivariate Gamma Function

The multivariate gamma function is defined as a multivariate extension of the gamma function. It is convenient for clearly expressing normalizing constants of matrix-variate distributions.

Definition 3.1 For $a > (p-1)/2$, the multivariate gamma function $\Gamma_p(a)$ is defined by

$$\Gamma_p(a) = \int_{\mathbb{S}_p^{(+)}} |\boldsymbol{W}|^{a-(p+1)/2} \exp(-\operatorname{tr} \boldsymbol{W})(\mathrm{d}\boldsymbol{W}).$$

When $p = 1$, $\Gamma(a) = \Gamma_1(a) = \int_0^\infty w^{a-1}e^{-w}\mathrm{d}w$, which is the usual gamma function. The multivariate gamma function can be rewritten as a product of the gamma functions.

Proposition 3.1 *For* $a > (p-1)/2$,

$$\Gamma_p(a) = \pi^{p(p-1)/4} \prod_{i=1}^{p} \Gamma\left(a - \frac{i-1}{2}\right).$$

Proof For $\boldsymbol{W} \in \mathbb{S}_p^{(+)}$, let $\boldsymbol{W} = \boldsymbol{T}\boldsymbol{T}^\top$ be the Cholesky decomposition of $\boldsymbol{W}$, where $\boldsymbol{T} = (t_{ij}) \in \mathbb{L}_p^{(+)}$. From Lemma 3.4, the Jacobian of transformation $\boldsymbol{W} \to \boldsymbol{T}$ is given by $J(\boldsymbol{W} \to \boldsymbol{T}) = 2^p \prod_{i=1}^p t_{ii}^{p-i+1}$, so that

$$\Gamma_p(a) = 2^p \int_{\mathbb{L}_p^{(+)}} |\boldsymbol{T}\boldsymbol{T}^\top|^{a-(p+1)/2} \exp(-\operatorname{tr} \boldsymbol{T}\boldsymbol{T}^\top) \left(\prod_{i=1}^{p} t_{ii}^{p-i+1}\right) (\mathrm{d}\boldsymbol{T}).$$

Since $|\boldsymbol{T}\boldsymbol{T}^\top| = \prod_{i=1}^p t_{ii}^2$ and $\operatorname{tr} \boldsymbol{T}\boldsymbol{T}^\top = \sum_{i=1}^p \sum_{j=1}^i t_{ij}^2$, we have

$$\begin{aligned}
\Gamma_p(a) &= 2^p \left(\prod_{i=2}^{p}\prod_{j=1}^{i-1} \int_{-\infty}^{\infty} e^{-t_{ij}^2}\mathrm{d}t_{ij}\right)\left(\prod_{i=1}^{p} \int_0^\infty t_{ii}^{2a-i} e^{-t_{ii}^2}\mathrm{d}t_{ii}\right) \\
&= 2^p \times (\sqrt{\pi})^{p(p-1)/2} \times \prod_{i=1}^{p} \frac{1}{2}\Gamma\left(a - \frac{i-1}{2}\right) \\
&= \pi^{p(p-1)/4} \prod_{i=1}^{p} \Gamma\left(a - \frac{i-1}{2}\right),
\end{aligned}$$

which completes the proof. □

3.2 The Matrix-Variate Normal Distribution

This section provides the definition of matrix-variate normal distribution and its useful properties to analyze a multivariate linear model. Here, the matrix-variate normal distribution is defined as an extension of $\mathcal{N}_p(\boldsymbol{\theta}, \boldsymbol{\Sigma})$.

Definition 3.2 For a random matrix $\boldsymbol{X} \in \mathbb{R}^{n\times p}$, assume that

$$\mathrm{vec}(\boldsymbol{X}^\top) \sim \mathcal{N}_{np}(\mathrm{vec}(\boldsymbol{M}^\top), \boldsymbol{\Omega} \otimes \boldsymbol{\Sigma}).$$

That is, $\mathrm{vec}(\boldsymbol{X}^\top)$ follows the (np)-variate normal distribution with mean $\mathrm{vec}(\boldsymbol{M}^\top)$ and covariance $\boldsymbol{\Omega} \otimes \boldsymbol{\Sigma}$, where $\boldsymbol{M} \in \mathbb{R}^{n\times p}$, and $\boldsymbol{\Omega} \in \mathbb{S}_n^{(+)}$ and $\boldsymbol{\Sigma} \in \mathbb{S}_p^{(+)}$. Then $\boldsymbol{X}$ is said to follow the matrix-variate normal distribution with mean matrix $\boldsymbol{M}$ and covariance matrix $\boldsymbol{\Omega} \otimes \boldsymbol{\Sigma}$, which is denoted by $\boldsymbol{X} \sim \mathcal{N}_{n\times p}(\boldsymbol{M}, \boldsymbol{\Omega} \otimes \boldsymbol{\Sigma})$.

Note that $\mathcal{N}_{np}(\boldsymbol{M}, \boldsymbol{\Omega} \otimes \boldsymbol{\Sigma})$ means an (np)-variate (vector-valued) normal distribution and is distinguished from $\mathcal{N}_{n\times p}(\boldsymbol{M}, \boldsymbol{\Omega} \otimes \boldsymbol{\Sigma})$.

The p.d.f. of the matrix-variate normal distribution can be written as follows.

Proposition 3.2 *The p.d.f. of $\mathcal{N}_{n\times p}(\boldsymbol{M}, \boldsymbol{\Omega} \otimes \boldsymbol{\Sigma})$ is given by*

$$\frac{1}{(2\pi)^{np/2}|\boldsymbol{\Omega}|^{p/2}|\boldsymbol{\Sigma}|^{n/2}} \exp\Big(-\frac{1}{2} \operatorname{tr} \boldsymbol{\Omega}^{-1}(\boldsymbol{X} - \boldsymbol{M})\boldsymbol{\Sigma}^{-1}(\boldsymbol{X} - \boldsymbol{M})^\top \Big).$$

Proof Using (iii) and (iv) of Lemma 2.4 and (ii) of Lemma 2.5, we observe $|\boldsymbol{\Omega} \otimes \boldsymbol{\Sigma}| = |\boldsymbol{\Omega}|^p |\boldsymbol{\Sigma}|^n$ and

$$\begin{aligned}
&\mathrm{vec}((\boldsymbol{X} - \boldsymbol{M})^\top)^\top (\boldsymbol{\Omega} \otimes \boldsymbol{\Sigma})^{-1} \mathrm{vec}((\boldsymbol{X} - \boldsymbol{M})^\top) \\
&= \mathrm{vec}((\boldsymbol{X} - \boldsymbol{M})^\top)^\top (\boldsymbol{\Omega}^{-1} \otimes \boldsymbol{\Sigma}^{-1}) \mathrm{vec}((\boldsymbol{X} - \boldsymbol{M})^\top) \\
&= \operatorname{tr} \boldsymbol{\Omega}^{-1}(\boldsymbol{X} - \boldsymbol{M})\boldsymbol{\Sigma}^{-1}(\boldsymbol{X} - \boldsymbol{M})^\top.
\end{aligned}$$

Since $\mathrm{vec}(\boldsymbol{X}^\top) \sim \mathcal{N}_{np}(\mathrm{vec}(\boldsymbol{M}^\top), \boldsymbol{\Omega} \otimes \boldsymbol{\Sigma})$, the p.d.f. is written as

$$\begin{aligned}
&\frac{1}{(2\pi)^{np/2}|\boldsymbol{\Omega} \otimes \boldsymbol{\Sigma}|^{1/2}} \exp\Big(-\frac{1}{2} \mathrm{vec}((\boldsymbol{X} - \boldsymbol{M})^\top)^\top (\boldsymbol{\Omega} \otimes \boldsymbol{\Sigma})^{-1} \mathrm{vec}((\boldsymbol{X} - \boldsymbol{M})^\top) \Big) \\
&= \frac{1}{(2\pi)^{np/2}|\boldsymbol{\Omega}|^{p/2}|\boldsymbol{\Sigma}|^{n/2}} \exp\Big(-\frac{1}{2} \operatorname{tr} \boldsymbol{\Omega}^{-1}(\boldsymbol{X} - \boldsymbol{M})\boldsymbol{\Sigma}^{-1}(\boldsymbol{X} - \boldsymbol{M})^\top \Big).
\end{aligned}$$

Hence the proof is complete. □

Using properties of the Kronecker product and the vec operator, we have the following proposition.

Proposition 3.3 *If $\boldsymbol{X} \sim \mathcal{N}_{n\times p}(\boldsymbol{M}, \boldsymbol{\Omega} \otimes \boldsymbol{\Sigma})$, then $\boldsymbol{X}^\top \sim \mathcal{N}_{p\times n}(\boldsymbol{M}^\top, \boldsymbol{\Sigma} \otimes \boldsymbol{\Omega})$.*

Proof Using (iv) of Lemma 2.4 and (ii) of Lemma 2.5 gives

$$\begin{aligned}\operatorname{tr}\boldsymbol{\Omega}^{-1}(\boldsymbol{X}-\boldsymbol{M})\boldsymbol{\Sigma}^{-1}(\boldsymbol{X}-\boldsymbol{M})^\top &= \operatorname{tr}\boldsymbol{\Sigma}^{-1}(\boldsymbol{X}-\boldsymbol{M})^\top\boldsymbol{\Omega}^{-1}(\boldsymbol{X}-\boldsymbol{M})\\ &= \operatorname{vec}(\boldsymbol{X}-\boldsymbol{M})^\top(\boldsymbol{\Sigma}\otimes\boldsymbol{\Omega})^{-1}\operatorname{vec}(\boldsymbol{X}-\boldsymbol{M}).\end{aligned}$$

This implies that $\operatorname{vec}(\boldsymbol{X}) \sim \mathcal{N}_{pn}(\operatorname{vec}(\boldsymbol{M}), \boldsymbol{\Sigma}\otimes\boldsymbol{\Omega})$. □

The first and second moments of the matrix-variate normal distribution are given in the following proposition.

Proposition 3.4 *Let* $\boldsymbol{X} = (x_{ij}) \sim \mathcal{N}_{n\times p}(\boldsymbol{M}, \boldsymbol{\Omega}\otimes\boldsymbol{\Sigma})$ *with* $\boldsymbol{M} = (\mu_{ij})$, $\boldsymbol{\Omega} = (\omega_{ij})$ *and* $\boldsymbol{\Sigma} = (\sigma_{ij})$*. Then, for any* $i, k \in \{1, \ldots, n\}$ *and* $j, l \in \{1, \ldots, p\}$,

$$E[x_{ij}] = \mu_{ij}, \qquad E[x_{ij}x_{kl}] = \omega_{ik}\sigma_{jl} + \mu_{ij}\mu_{kl}.$$

Proof Let $\boldsymbol{X} = (\boldsymbol{x}_1, \ldots, \boldsymbol{x}_n)^\top$ and $\boldsymbol{M} = (\boldsymbol{\mu}_1, \ldots, \boldsymbol{\mu}_n)^\top$, where $\boldsymbol{x}_i = (x_{i1}, \ldots, x_{ip})^\top \in \mathbb{R}^p$ and $\boldsymbol{\mu}_i = (\mu_{i1}, \ldots, \mu_{ip})^\top \in \mathbb{R}^p$ for $i = 1, \ldots, n$. Then

$$\operatorname{vec}(\boldsymbol{X}^\top) = \begin{pmatrix}\boldsymbol{x}_1\\ \vdots\\ \boldsymbol{x}_n\end{pmatrix} \sim \mathcal{N}_{np}\left(\begin{pmatrix}\boldsymbol{\mu}_1\\ \vdots\\ \boldsymbol{\mu}_n\end{pmatrix}, \begin{pmatrix}\omega_{11}\boldsymbol{\Sigma} & \ldots & \omega_{1n}\boldsymbol{\Sigma}\\ \vdots & & \vdots\\ \omega_{n1}\boldsymbol{\Sigma} & \ldots & \omega_{nn}\boldsymbol{\Sigma}\end{pmatrix}\right),$$

implying that, according to (i) of Lemma 3.1,

$$E[\boldsymbol{x}_i] = \boldsymbol{\mu}_i, \quad E[(\boldsymbol{x}_i - \boldsymbol{\mu}_i)(\boldsymbol{x}_k - \boldsymbol{\mu}_k)^\top] = \omega_{ik}\boldsymbol{\Sigma},$$

further implying that

$$E[x_{ij}] = \mu_{ij}, \qquad E[(x_{ij} - \mu_{ij})(x_{kl} - \mu_{kl})] = \omega_{ik}\sigma_{jl}.$$

Hence the proof is complete. □

Proposition 3.4 suggests that, if $\boldsymbol{X} \sim \mathcal{N}_{n\times p}(\boldsymbol{M}, \boldsymbol{\Omega}\otimes\boldsymbol{\Sigma})$, covariance of any two rows of $\boldsymbol{X}$ is proportional to $\boldsymbol{\Sigma}$ and also covariance of any two columns of $\boldsymbol{X}$ is proportional to $\boldsymbol{\Omega}$. Further Proposition 3.4 yields the following corollary.

Corollary 3.1 *If* $\boldsymbol{X} \sim \mathcal{N}_{n\times p}(\boldsymbol{M}, \boldsymbol{\Omega}\otimes\boldsymbol{\Sigma})$*, then*

$$\begin{aligned}E[\boldsymbol{X}] &= \boldsymbol{M},\\ E[\boldsymbol{X}^\top\boldsymbol{A}\boldsymbol{X}] &= (\operatorname{tr}\boldsymbol{A}\boldsymbol{\Omega})\boldsymbol{\Sigma} + \boldsymbol{M}^\top\boldsymbol{A}\boldsymbol{M},\\ E[\boldsymbol{X}\boldsymbol{B}\boldsymbol{X}^\top] &= (\operatorname{tr}\boldsymbol{B}\boldsymbol{\Sigma})\boldsymbol{\Omega} + \boldsymbol{M}\boldsymbol{B}\boldsymbol{M}^\top\end{aligned}$$

for constant matrices $\boldsymbol{A} \in \mathbb{R}^{n\times n}$ *and* $\boldsymbol{B} \in \mathbb{R}^{p\times p}$.

Proof Using Proposition 3.4 immediately gives $E[\boldsymbol{X}] = (E[x_{ij}]) = (\mu_{ij}) = \boldsymbol{M}$. Let $\boldsymbol{A} = (a_{ij})$ and $\boldsymbol{B} = (b_{ij})$. For $i, j \in \{1, \ldots, p\}$, the (i, j)-th element of $\boldsymbol{X}^\top \boldsymbol{A}\boldsymbol{X}$ is $\{\boldsymbol{X}^\top \boldsymbol{A}\boldsymbol{X}\}_{ij} = \sum_{k=1}^n \sum_{l=1}^n x_{ki}a_{kl}x_{lj}$, so that

$$\begin{aligned}E[\{\boldsymbol{X}^\top \boldsymbol{A}\boldsymbol{X}\}_{ij}] &= \sum_{k=1}^n \sum_{l=1}^n a_{kl}E[x_{ki}x_{lj}] \\ &= \sum_{k=1}^n \sum_{l=1}^n a_{kl}(\omega_{kl}\sigma_{ij} + \mu_{ki}\mu_{lj}) \\ &= (\operatorname{tr} \boldsymbol{A}\boldsymbol{\Omega}^\top)\sigma_{ij} + \{\boldsymbol{M}^\top \boldsymbol{A}\boldsymbol{M}\}_{ij}.\end{aligned}$$

It holds that $\operatorname{tr} \boldsymbol{A}\boldsymbol{\Omega}^\top = \operatorname{tr} \boldsymbol{A}\boldsymbol{\Omega}$, so that $E[\boldsymbol{X}^\top \boldsymbol{A}\boldsymbol{X}] = (\operatorname{tr} \boldsymbol{A}\boldsymbol{\Omega})\boldsymbol{\Sigma} + \boldsymbol{M}^\top \boldsymbol{A}\boldsymbol{M}$. Similarly, for $i, j \in \{1, \ldots, n\}$,

$$\begin{aligned}E[\{\boldsymbol{X}\boldsymbol{B}\boldsymbol{X}^\top\}_{ij}] &= \sum_{k=1}^p \sum_{l=1}^p b_{kl}E[x_{ik}x_{jl}] \\ &= \sum_{k=1}^p \sum_{l=1}^p b_{kl}(\omega_{ij}\sigma_{kl} + \mu_{ik}\mu_{jl}) \\ &= (\operatorname{tr} \boldsymbol{B}\boldsymbol{\Sigma})\omega_{ij} + \{\boldsymbol{M}\boldsymbol{B}\boldsymbol{M}^\top\}_{ij}.\end{aligned}$$

Hence the proof is complete. □

Next, we provide a result on linear transformation of the matrix-variate normal distribution. The following proposition is an extension of (ii) in Lemma 3.1.

Proposition 3.5 *Let* $\boldsymbol{A}$ *be a full row rank constant matrix in* $\mathbb{R}^{m\times n}$ *and let* $\boldsymbol{B}$ *be a full column rank constant matrix in* $\mathbb{R}^{p\times q}$*. Also, let* $\boldsymbol{C}$ *be a constant matrix in* $\mathbb{R}^{m\times q}$*. If* $\boldsymbol{X} \sim \mathcal{N}_{n\times p}(\boldsymbol{M}, \boldsymbol{\Omega} \otimes \boldsymbol{\Sigma})$*, then*

$$\boldsymbol{A}\boldsymbol{X}\boldsymbol{B} + \boldsymbol{C} \sim \mathcal{N}_{m\times q}(\boldsymbol{A}\boldsymbol{M}\boldsymbol{B} + \boldsymbol{C}, \boldsymbol{A}\boldsymbol{\Omega}\boldsymbol{A}^\top \otimes \boldsymbol{B}^\top \boldsymbol{\Sigma}\boldsymbol{B}).$$

Proof From (i) of Lemma 2.5, it is seen that $\operatorname{vec}((\boldsymbol{A}\boldsymbol{X}\boldsymbol{B} + \boldsymbol{C})^\top) = \operatorname{vec}(\boldsymbol{B}^\top \boldsymbol{X}^\top \boldsymbol{A}^\top) + \operatorname{vec}(\boldsymbol{C}^\top) = (\boldsymbol{A} \otimes \boldsymbol{B}^\top)\operatorname{vec}(\boldsymbol{X}^\top) + \operatorname{vec}(\boldsymbol{C}^\top)$. Using (ii) of Lemma 3.1 gives

$$\begin{aligned}&(\boldsymbol{A} \otimes \boldsymbol{B}^\top)\operatorname{vec}(\boldsymbol{X}^\top) + \operatorname{vec}(\boldsymbol{C}^\top) \\ &\sim \mathcal{N}_{mq}((\boldsymbol{A} \otimes \boldsymbol{B}^\top)\operatorname{vec}(\boldsymbol{M}^\top) + \operatorname{vec}(\boldsymbol{C}^\top), (\boldsymbol{A} \otimes \boldsymbol{B}^\top)(\boldsymbol{\Omega} \otimes \boldsymbol{\Sigma})(\boldsymbol{A} \otimes \boldsymbol{B}^\top)^\top),\end{aligned}$$

which implies from (i) and (ii) of Lemma 2.4 that

$$(\boldsymbol{A} \otimes \boldsymbol{B}^\top)\operatorname{vec}(\boldsymbol{X}^\top) + \operatorname{vec}(\boldsymbol{C}^\top) \sim \mathcal{N}_{mq}(\operatorname{vec}((\boldsymbol{A}\boldsymbol{M}\boldsymbol{B} + \boldsymbol{C})^\top), \boldsymbol{A}\boldsymbol{\Omega}\boldsymbol{A}^\top \otimes \boldsymbol{B}^\top \boldsymbol{\Sigma}\boldsymbol{B}).$$

Hence the proof is complete. □

A partitioning of a random matrix is needed in various fields of statistical inference. Here we give a distributional property for a partitioned random matrix with respect to the matrix-variate normal distribution. The following proposition is a generalization from (iii) of Lemma 3.1.

Proposition 3.6 *Let* $\boldsymbol{X} \sim \mathcal{N}_{n\times p}(\boldsymbol{M}, \boldsymbol{\Omega} \otimes \boldsymbol{\Sigma})$. *Partition* $\boldsymbol{X}$, $\boldsymbol{M}$ *and* $\boldsymbol{\Omega}$ *as, respectively,*

$$\boldsymbol{X} = \begin{pmatrix} \boldsymbol{X}_1 \\ \boldsymbol{X}_2 \end{pmatrix}, \quad \boldsymbol{M} = \begin{pmatrix} \boldsymbol{M}_1 \\ \boldsymbol{M}_2 \end{pmatrix} \quad \text{and} \quad \boldsymbol{\Omega} = \begin{pmatrix} \boldsymbol{\Omega}_{11} & \boldsymbol{\Omega}_{21}^\top \\ \boldsymbol{\Omega}_{21} & \boldsymbol{\Omega}_{22} \end{pmatrix},$$

where $\boldsymbol{X}_1 \in \mathbb{R}^{m\times p}$, $\boldsymbol{M}_1 \in \mathbb{R}^{m\times p}$ *and* $\boldsymbol{\Omega}_{11} \in \mathbb{S}_m^{(+)}$. *Let* $\boldsymbol{\Omega}_{22\cdot 1} = \boldsymbol{\Omega}_{22} - \boldsymbol{\Omega}_{21}\boldsymbol{\Omega}_{11}^{-1}\boldsymbol{\Omega}_{21}^\top$. *Then*

$$\begin{aligned} \boldsymbol{X}_1 &\sim \mathcal{N}_{m\times p}(\boldsymbol{M}_1, \boldsymbol{\Omega}_{11} \otimes \boldsymbol{\Sigma}), \\ \boldsymbol{X}_2|\boldsymbol{X}_1 &\sim \mathcal{N}_{(n-m)\times p}(\boldsymbol{M}_2 + \boldsymbol{\Omega}_{21}\boldsymbol{\Omega}_{11}^{-1}(\boldsymbol{X}_1 - \boldsymbol{M}_1), \boldsymbol{\Omega}_{22\cdot 1} \otimes \boldsymbol{\Sigma}). \end{aligned}$$

Further, if $\boldsymbol{\Omega}_{21} = \boldsymbol{0}_{(n-m)\times m}$ *then* $\boldsymbol{X}_1$ *and* $\boldsymbol{X}_2$ *are independently distributed as* $\boldsymbol{X}_1 \sim \mathcal{N}_{m\times p}(\boldsymbol{M}_1, \boldsymbol{\Omega}_{11} \otimes \boldsymbol{\Sigma})$ *and* $\boldsymbol{X}_2 \sim \mathcal{N}_{(n-m)\times p}(\boldsymbol{M}_2, \boldsymbol{\Omega}_{22} \otimes \boldsymbol{\Sigma})$.

Proof Lemma 2.1 guarantees $\boldsymbol{\Omega}_{11}$ and $\boldsymbol{\Omega}_{22\cdot 1}$ to be nonsingular. Using (2.1) gives that $|\boldsymbol{\Omega}| = |\boldsymbol{\Omega}_{11}| \times |\boldsymbol{\Omega}_{22\cdot 1}|$ and

$$\boldsymbol{\Omega}^{-1} = \begin{pmatrix} \boldsymbol{I}_m & -\boldsymbol{\Omega}_{11}^{-1}\boldsymbol{\Omega}_{21}^\top \\ \boldsymbol{0}_{(n-m)\times m} & \boldsymbol{I}_{n-m} \end{pmatrix} \begin{pmatrix} \boldsymbol{\Omega}_{11}^{-1} & \boldsymbol{0}_{m\times(n-m)} \\ \boldsymbol{0}_{(n-m)\times m} & \boldsymbol{\Omega}_{22\cdot 1}^{-1} \end{pmatrix} \begin{pmatrix} \boldsymbol{I}_m & \boldsymbol{0}_{m\times(n-m)} \\ -\boldsymbol{\Omega}_{21}\boldsymbol{\Omega}_{11}^{-1} & \boldsymbol{I}_{n-m} \end{pmatrix}.$$

Here, $(\boldsymbol{X} - \boldsymbol{M})^\top \boldsymbol{\Omega}^{-1}(\boldsymbol{X} - \boldsymbol{M})$ becomes

$$\begin{aligned} &(\boldsymbol{X}_1 - \boldsymbol{M}_1)^\top \boldsymbol{\Omega}_{11}^{-1}(\boldsymbol{X}_1 - \boldsymbol{M}_1) \\ &\quad + \{\boldsymbol{X}_2 - \boldsymbol{M}_2 - \boldsymbol{\Omega}_{21}\boldsymbol{\Omega}_{11}^{-1}(\boldsymbol{X}_1 - \boldsymbol{M}_1)\}^\top \boldsymbol{\Omega}_{22\cdot 1}^{-1}\{\boldsymbol{X}_2 - \boldsymbol{M}_2 - \boldsymbol{\Omega}_{21}\boldsymbol{\Omega}_{11}^{-1}(\boldsymbol{X}_1 - \boldsymbol{M}_1)\}. \end{aligned}$$

From Proposition 3.2, the p.d.f. of $\boldsymbol{X}$ is rewritten as

$$\begin{aligned} &c_1 \exp\Big(-\frac{1}{2} \operatorname{tr} \boldsymbol{\Omega}_{11}^{-1}(\boldsymbol{X}_1 - \boldsymbol{M}_1)\boldsymbol{\Sigma}^{-1}(\boldsymbol{X}_1 - \boldsymbol{M}_1)^\top \Big) \\ &\times c_2 \exp\Big(-\frac{1}{2} \operatorname{tr} \boldsymbol{\Omega}_{22\cdot 1}^{-1}\{\boldsymbol{X}_2 - \boldsymbol{M}_2 - \boldsymbol{\Omega}_{21}\boldsymbol{\Omega}_{11}^{-1}(\boldsymbol{X}_1 - \boldsymbol{M}_1)\} \\ &\qquad \times \boldsymbol{\Sigma}^{-1}\{\boldsymbol{X}_2 - \boldsymbol{M}_2 - \boldsymbol{\Omega}_{21}\boldsymbol{\Omega}_{11}^{-1}(\boldsymbol{X}_1 - \boldsymbol{M}_1)\}^\top \Big), \end{aligned}$$

where

$$c_1 = (2\pi)^{-mp/2}|\boldsymbol{\Omega}_{11}|^{-p/2}|\boldsymbol{\Sigma}|^{-m/2}, \quad c_2 = (2\pi)^{-(n-m)p/2}|\boldsymbol{\Omega}_{22\cdot 1}|^{-p/2}|\boldsymbol{\Sigma}|^{-(n-m)/2}.$$

Hence the above joint p.d.f. of $\boldsymbol{X}_1$ and $\boldsymbol{X}_2$ suggests that $\boldsymbol{X}_1 \sim \mathcal{N}_{m\times p}(\boldsymbol{M}_1, \boldsymbol{\Omega}_{11} \otimes \boldsymbol{\Sigma})$ and $\boldsymbol{X}_2|\boldsymbol{X}_1 \sim \mathcal{N}_{(n-m)\times p}(\boldsymbol{M}_2 + \boldsymbol{\Omega}_{21}\boldsymbol{\Omega}_{11}^{-1}(\boldsymbol{X}_1 - \boldsymbol{M}_1), \boldsymbol{\Omega}_{22\cdot 1} \otimes \boldsymbol{\Sigma})$.

When $\boldsymbol{\Omega}_{21} = \mathbf{0}_{(n-m)\times m}$, it is seen that $\boldsymbol{\Omega}_{22\cdot 1} = \boldsymbol{\Omega}_{22}$ and $\boldsymbol{X}_2 \sim \mathcal{N}_{(n-m)\times p}(\boldsymbol{M}_2, \boldsymbol{\Omega}_{22} \otimes \boldsymbol{\Sigma})$. As a consequence, $\boldsymbol{X}_2$ does not depend on $\boldsymbol{X}_1$, and thus $\boldsymbol{X}_1$ and $\boldsymbol{X}_2$ are mutually independent. □

Proposition 3.6 suggests that if $\boldsymbol{X} \sim \mathcal{N}_{n\times p}(\boldsymbol{M}, \boldsymbol{\Omega} \otimes \boldsymbol{\Sigma})$ and $\boldsymbol{\Omega}$ is a diagonal matrix then all the rows of $\boldsymbol{X}$ are mutually independent.

Various properties of the matrix-variate normal distribution have been discovered and studied in addition to useful properties mentioned above. For other properties of the matrix-variate normal distribution, see Gupta and Nagar (1999) and Muirhead (1982).

3.3 The Wishart Distribution

The Wishart distribution is known as a distribution of the sample covariance matrix in a multivariate normal model and plays an important role in multivariate analysis. It is named for Wishart (1928). First, we provide the definition of the Wishart distribution.

Definition 3.3 Let $\boldsymbol{X} \sim \mathcal{N}_{n\times p}(\mathbf{0}_{n\times p}, \boldsymbol{I}_n \otimes \boldsymbol{\Sigma})$ with $\boldsymbol{\Sigma} \in \mathbb{S}_p^{(+)}$ and denote $\nu = n \wedge p$. Then $\boldsymbol{S} = \boldsymbol{X}^\top \boldsymbol{X}$ is called the Wishart matrix of rank ν and is said to follow the Wishart distribution with n degrees of freedom and scale matrix $\boldsymbol{\Sigma}$, which is denoted by $\boldsymbol{S} \sim \mathcal{W}_p^\nu(n, \boldsymbol{\Sigma})$.

If $n \ge p$, $\mathcal{W}_p^p(n, \boldsymbol{\Sigma})$ is often abbreviated to $\mathcal{W}_p(n, \boldsymbol{\Sigma})$ and the Wishart matrix $\boldsymbol{S}$ lies in $\mathbb{S}_p^{(+)}$ with probability one.

When $p > n$, the Wishart matrix is singular with probability one and belongs to $\mathbb{S}_{p,n}^{(+)}$. Then in the literature, the distribution of the Wishart matrix is called a pseudo-Wishart distribution. See Srivastava and Khatri (1979) and Díaz-García et al. (1997).

The following proposition provides a unified p.d.f. of $\mathcal{W}_p^\nu(n, \boldsymbol{\Sigma})$ in the nonsingular and the singular cases of the Wishart matrix.

Proposition 3.7 *Let* $(\mathrm{d}\boldsymbol{S})$ *be defined as in Lemma 3.5 with* $r = \nu$. *The p.d.f. of* $\mathcal{W}_p^\nu(n, \boldsymbol{\Sigma})$ *with respect to* $(\mathrm{d}\boldsymbol{S})$ *is expressed by*

$$\frac{\pi^{n(\nu-p)/2}}{2^{np/2}|\boldsymbol{\Sigma}|^{n/2}\Gamma_\nu(n/2)}|\boldsymbol{L}|^{(n-p-1)/2}\exp\Big(-\frac{1}{2}\operatorname{tr}\boldsymbol{\Sigma}^{-1}\boldsymbol{S}\Big),$$

where $\boldsymbol{L} \in \mathbb{D}_\nu^{(\ge 0)}$ *and the diagonal of* $\boldsymbol{L}$ *consists of* ν *positive eigenvalues of* $\boldsymbol{S}$.

Proof Let $\boldsymbol{X} = (x_{ij}) \sim \mathcal{N}_{n\times p}(\mathbf{0}_{n\times p}, \boldsymbol{I}_n \otimes \boldsymbol{\Sigma})$. Note from Proposition 3.3 that $\boldsymbol{X}^\top \sim \mathcal{N}_{p\times n}(\mathbf{0}_{p\times n}, \boldsymbol{\Sigma} \otimes \boldsymbol{I}_n)$. Let $\boldsymbol{X}^\top = \boldsymbol{V}\boldsymbol{D}\boldsymbol{U}^\top$ be the singular value decomposition of $\boldsymbol{X}^\top$, where $\boldsymbol{V} \in \mathbb{V}_{p,\nu}$, $\boldsymbol{D} = \operatorname{diag}(d_1, \ldots, d_\nu) \in \mathbb{D}_\nu^{(\ge 0)}$ and $\boldsymbol{U} \in \mathbb{V}_{n,\nu}$. Since the p.d.f. of $\mathcal{N}_{p\times n}(\mathbf{0}_{p\times n}, \boldsymbol{\Sigma} \otimes \boldsymbol{I}_n)$ with respect to $(\mathrm{d}\boldsymbol{X}^\top) = \bigwedge_{j=1}^p \bigwedge_{i=1}^n \mathrm{d}x_{ij}$ on $\mathbb{R}^{p\times n}$ is given by

$$\frac{1}{(2\pi)^{np/2}|\boldsymbol{\Sigma}|^{n/2}}\exp\Big(-\frac{1}{2}\operatorname{tr}\boldsymbol{\Sigma}^{-1}\boldsymbol{X}^\top\boldsymbol{X}\Big)(\mathrm{d}\boldsymbol{X}^\top). \tag{3.2}$$

Lemma 3.6 is used to express the joint (unnormalized) p.d.f. of $\boldsymbol{V}$, $\boldsymbol{D}$ and $\boldsymbol{U}$ as

$$\frac{1}{(2\pi)^{np/2}|\boldsymbol{\Sigma}|^{n/2}} \exp\Big(-\frac{1}{2}\operatorname{tr}\boldsymbol{\Sigma}^{-1}\boldsymbol{V}\boldsymbol{D}^2\boldsymbol{V}^\top\Big) \times 2^{-\nu}|\boldsymbol{D}|^{n+p-2\nu}\left(\prod_{1\le i<j\le\nu}(d_i^2-d_j^2)\right)(\boldsymbol{V}^\top \mathrm{d}\boldsymbol{V})(\mathrm{d}\boldsymbol{D})(\boldsymbol{U}^\top \mathrm{d}\boldsymbol{U}).$$

Note from (3.1) that $\int_{\mathbb{V}_{n,\nu}}(\boldsymbol{U}^\top \mathrm{d}\boldsymbol{U}) = 2^\nu\pi^{n\nu/2}/\Gamma_\nu(n/2)$. Making the transformation $\boldsymbol{L} = \operatorname{diag}(\ell_1,\ldots,\ell_\nu) = \boldsymbol{D}^2$ and integrating out with respect to $\boldsymbol{U}$, we obtain the joint (unnormalized) p.d.f. of $\boldsymbol{V}$ and $\boldsymbol{L}$:

$$\frac{\pi^{n\nu/2}}{(2\pi)^{np/2}|\boldsymbol{\Sigma}|^{n/2}\Gamma_\nu(n/2)} \exp\Big(-\frac{1}{2}\operatorname{tr}\boldsymbol{\Sigma}^{-1}\boldsymbol{V}\boldsymbol{L}\boldsymbol{V}^\top\Big) \times 2^{-\nu}|\boldsymbol{L}|^{(n+p-2\nu-1)/2}\left(\prod_{1\le i<j\le\nu}(\ell_i-\ell_j)\right)(\boldsymbol{V}^\top \mathrm{d}\boldsymbol{V})(\mathrm{d}\boldsymbol{L}). \tag{3.3}$$

Let $\boldsymbol{S} = \boldsymbol{X}^\top\boldsymbol{X} = \boldsymbol{V}\boldsymbol{L}\boldsymbol{V}^\top$. From Lemma 3.5,

$$(\mathrm{d}\boldsymbol{S}) = \frac{1}{2^\nu}|\boldsymbol{L}|^{p-\nu}\left(\prod_{1\le i<j\le\nu}(\ell_i-\ell_j)\right)(\mathrm{d}\boldsymbol{L})(\boldsymbol{V}^\top \mathrm{d}\boldsymbol{V}),$$

which yields the p.d.f. of $\boldsymbol{S}$. □

Equation (3.3) is the joint (unnormalized) p.d.f. of nonzero eigenvalues and the corresponding eigenvectors for the Wishart matrix $\boldsymbol{S} \in \mathbb{S}_{p,\nu}^{(+)}$. Note that, for $\nu = p$, $\boldsymbol{S} \in \mathbb{S}_p^{(+)}$ and then the p.d.f. of $\mathcal{W}_p(n, \boldsymbol{\Sigma})$ on $\mathbb{S}_p^{(+)}$ can be expressed as

$$\frac{1}{2^{np/2}|\boldsymbol{\Sigma}|^{n/2}\Gamma_p(n/2)}|\boldsymbol{S}|^{(n-p-1)/2}\exp\Big(-\frac{1}{2}\operatorname{tr}\boldsymbol{\Sigma}^{-1}\boldsymbol{S}\Big),$$

because $|\boldsymbol{L}| = |\boldsymbol{S}|$ in Proposition 3.7. When $p = 1$ and $\boldsymbol{\Sigma} = 1$, the p.d.f. above is the same as that of the chi-square distribution with n degrees of freedom. Thus the Wishart distribution is a multivariate generalization of the chi-square distribution.

The following proposition is an important result on expectation of the Wishart matrix, which is the basis for unbiased estimation of $\boldsymbol{\Sigma}$.

Proposition 3.8 *Let* $\boldsymbol{S} \sim \mathcal{W}_p^\nu(n, \boldsymbol{\Sigma})$. *Then* $E[\boldsymbol{S}] = n\boldsymbol{\Sigma}$.

Proof Recall that $\boldsymbol{S} = \boldsymbol{X}^\top\boldsymbol{X}$, where $\boldsymbol{X} \sim \mathcal{N}_{n\times p}(\boldsymbol{0}_{n\times p}, \boldsymbol{I}_n \otimes \boldsymbol{\Sigma})$. Thus, this proposition can immediately be verified by Corollary 3.1. □

From Proposition 3.8, $\mathcal{W}_p^\nu(n, \boldsymbol{\Sigma})$ is also called the Wishart distribution with n degrees of freedom and mean $n\boldsymbol{\Sigma}$.

Many interesting results on the Wishart distribution have already been obtained in the literature. For other results on the Wishart distribution, see Gupta and Nagar (1999) and Muirhead (1982).

3.4 The Cholesky Decomposition of the Wishart Matrix

Here, we provide distribution theories related to the Cholesky decomposition of the Wishart matrix. This decomposition is also named the Bartlett decomposition in statistics.

Let $\boldsymbol{X} = (x_{ij}) \sim \mathcal{N}_{n\times p}(\mathbf{0}_{n\times p}, \boldsymbol{I}_n \otimes \boldsymbol{\Sigma})$. The Wishart matrix is defined by $\boldsymbol{S} = \boldsymbol{X}^\top \boldsymbol{X}$. In the case of $p > n$, partition $\boldsymbol{X}$ as $\boldsymbol{X} = (\boldsymbol{X}_1^\top, \boldsymbol{X}_2^\top)$, where $\boldsymbol{X}_1 \in \mathbb{R}^{n\times n}$, and denote by $\boldsymbol{X}_1 = \boldsymbol{T}_1 \boldsymbol{Q}^\top$ uniquely the LQ decomposition of $\boldsymbol{X}_1$, where $\boldsymbol{T}_1 \in \mathbb{L}_n^{(+)}$ and $\boldsymbol{Q} \in \mathbb{O}_n$. Here,

$$\boldsymbol{X}^\top = \begin{pmatrix} \boldsymbol{X}_1 \\ \boldsymbol{X}_2 \end{pmatrix} = \begin{pmatrix} \boldsymbol{T}_1 \boldsymbol{Q}^\top \\ \boldsymbol{X}_2 \end{pmatrix} = \begin{pmatrix} \boldsymbol{T}_1 \\ \boldsymbol{X}_2 \boldsymbol{Q} \end{pmatrix} \boldsymbol{Q}^\top \equiv \boldsymbol{T}\boldsymbol{Q}^\top, \tag{3.4}$$

where $\boldsymbol{T} = (\boldsymbol{T}_1^\top, \boldsymbol{T}_2^\top)^\top \in \mathbb{L}_{p,n}^{(+)}$ and $\boldsymbol{T}_2 = \boldsymbol{X}_2 \boldsymbol{Q} \in \mathbb{R}^{(p-n)\times n}$, which yields $\boldsymbol{S} = \boldsymbol{T}\boldsymbol{T}^\top$. When $n \ge p$, the usual Cholesky decomposition of $\boldsymbol{S}$ is given by $\boldsymbol{S} = \boldsymbol{T}\boldsymbol{T}^\top$, where $\boldsymbol{T} \in \mathbb{L}_p^{(+)} = \mathbb{L}_{p,p}^{(+)}$. Hence the above decompositions for the cases of $n \ge p$ and $p > n$ can be integrated into $\boldsymbol{S} = \boldsymbol{T}\boldsymbol{T}^\top$, where a unique $\boldsymbol{T} \in \mathbb{L}_{p,\nu}^{(+)}$ with $\nu = n \wedge p$. Then we have the following proposition.

Proposition 3.9 *The p.d.f. of* $\boldsymbol{T} = (t_{ij}) \in \mathbb{L}_{p,\nu}^{(+)}$ *with* $\nu = n \wedge p$ *is given by*

$$\frac{2^\nu \pi^{n\nu/2}}{(2\pi)^{np/2} |\boldsymbol{\Sigma}|^{n/2} \Gamma_\nu(n/2)} \exp\Big(-\frac{1}{2} \operatorname{tr} \boldsymbol{\Sigma}^{-1} \boldsymbol{T}\boldsymbol{T}^\top \Big) \prod_{i=1}^{\nu} t_{ii}^{n-i}. \tag{3.5}$$

Proof For the $n \ge p$ case, let $\boldsymbol{X}^\top = \boldsymbol{T}\boldsymbol{Q}^\top$ be the LQ decomposition of $\boldsymbol{X}^\top$, where $\boldsymbol{T} \in \mathbb{L}_p^{(+)}$ and $\boldsymbol{Q} \in \mathbb{V}_{n,p}$. Making the transformation $\boldsymbol{X}^\top \to (\boldsymbol{T}, \boldsymbol{Q})$ in (3.2) and using Lemma 3.3, we can write the joint (unnormalized) p.d.f. of $\boldsymbol{T}$ and $\boldsymbol{Q}$ as

$$\frac{1}{(2\pi)^{np/2} |\boldsymbol{\Sigma}|^{n/2}} \exp\Big(-\frac{1}{2} \operatorname{tr} \boldsymbol{\Sigma}^{-1} \boldsymbol{T}\boldsymbol{T}^\top \Big) \Big(\prod_{i=1}^{p} t_{ii}^{n-i} \Big) (\mathrm{d}\boldsymbol{T})(\boldsymbol{Q}^\top \mathrm{d}\boldsymbol{Q}).$$

From (3.1), integrating out with respect to $\boldsymbol{Q}$ gives

$$\frac{2^p \pi^{np/2}}{(2\pi)^{np/2} |\boldsymbol{\Sigma}|^{n/2} \Gamma_p(n/2)} \exp\Big(-\frac{1}{2} \operatorname{tr} \boldsymbol{\Sigma}^{-1} \boldsymbol{T}\boldsymbol{T}^\top \Big) \Big(\prod_{i=1}^{p} t_{ii}^{n-i} \Big) (\mathrm{d}\boldsymbol{T}).$$

This is the p.d.f. of $\boldsymbol{T}$ for the $n \ge p$ case.

When $p > n$, noting from (3.4) that $(\mathrm{d}\boldsymbol{X}_2) = (\mathrm{d}\boldsymbol{T}_2)$, we see

$$(\mathrm{d}\boldsymbol{X}^\top) = (\mathrm{d}\boldsymbol{X}_1)(\mathrm{d}\boldsymbol{X}_2) = \left(\prod_{i=1}^{n} t_{ii}^{n-i}\right)(\mathrm{d}\boldsymbol{T}_1)(\boldsymbol{Q}^\top \mathrm{d}\boldsymbol{Q})(\mathrm{d}\boldsymbol{X}_2) = \left(\prod_{i=1}^{n} t_{ii}^{n-i}\right)(\mathrm{d}\boldsymbol{T})(\boldsymbol{Q}^\top \mathrm{d}\boldsymbol{Q}).$$

Hence the joint (unnormalized) p.d.f. of $\boldsymbol{T} \in \mathbb{L}_n^{(+)}$ and $\boldsymbol{Q} \in \mathbb{O}_n = \mathbb{V}_{n,n}$ can be expressed as

$$\frac{1}{(2\pi)^{np/2}|\boldsymbol{\Sigma}|^{n/2}} \exp\left(-\frac{1}{2}\operatorname{tr}\boldsymbol{\Sigma}^{-1}\boldsymbol{T}\boldsymbol{T}^\top\right)\left(\prod_{i=1}^{n} t_{ii}^{n-i}\right)(\mathrm{d}\boldsymbol{T})(\boldsymbol{Q}^\top \mathrm{d}\boldsymbol{Q}).$$

Using (3.1) gives $\int_{\mathbb{V}_{n,n}}(\boldsymbol{Q}^\top \mathrm{d}\boldsymbol{Q}) = 2^n\pi^{n^2/2}/\Gamma_n(n/2)$, yielding the p.d.f. of $\boldsymbol{T}$ given in (3.5) with $\nu = n$. □

For deriving moments of $\boldsymbol{T}$, we provide the distributions of nonzero elements in each column of $\boldsymbol{T}$. Define the Cholesky decomposition of $\boldsymbol{\Sigma}$ as $\boldsymbol{\Sigma} = \boldsymbol{\Xi}\boldsymbol{\Xi}^\top$, where $\boldsymbol{\Xi} = (\xi_{i,j}) \in \mathbb{L}_p^{(+)}$. Denote $\boldsymbol{\Xi}_{(1)} = \boldsymbol{\Xi}$, $\boldsymbol{\Xi}_{(p)} = \xi_{p,p}$ and, for $i = 1, \ldots, p-1$,

$$\boldsymbol{\Xi}_{(i)} = \begin{pmatrix} \xi_{i,i} & \boldsymbol{0}_{p-i}^\top \\ \boldsymbol{\xi}_{(i)} & \boldsymbol{\Xi}_{(i+1)} \end{pmatrix} \in \mathbb{L}_{p-i+1}^{(+)},$$

where

$$\boldsymbol{\xi}_{(i)} = \begin{pmatrix} \xi_{i+1,i} \\ \vdots \\ \xi_{p,i} \end{pmatrix} \in \mathbb{R}^{p-i}, \quad \boldsymbol{\Xi}_{(i+1)} = \begin{pmatrix} \xi_{i+1,i+1} & & 0 \\ \vdots & \ddots & \\ \xi_{p,i+1} & \cdots & \xi_{p,p} \end{pmatrix} \in \mathbb{L}_{p-i}^{(+)}.$$

Let $\boldsymbol{\gamma}_{(i)} = (\gamma_{i+1,i}, \ldots, \gamma_{p,i})^\top = \xi_{i,i}^{-1}\boldsymbol{\xi}_{(i)}$ for $i = 1, \ldots, p-1$ and let $\sigma_i^2 = \xi_{i,i}^2$ for $i = 1, \ldots, p$. For $i = 1, \ldots, p$, let $\boldsymbol{\Sigma}_{(i)} = \boldsymbol{\Xi}_{(i)}\boldsymbol{\Xi}_{(i)}^\top$, where $\boldsymbol{\Sigma}_{(1)} = \boldsymbol{\Sigma}$ and $\boldsymbol{\Sigma}_{(p)} = \sigma_p^2$. Note that for $i = 1, \ldots, p-1$

$$\boldsymbol{\Sigma}_{(i)} = \begin{pmatrix} 1 & \boldsymbol{0}_{p-i}^\top \\ \boldsymbol{\gamma}_{(i)} & \boldsymbol{I}_{p-i} \end{pmatrix} \begin{pmatrix} \sigma_i^2 & \boldsymbol{0}_{p-i}^\top \\ \boldsymbol{0}_{p-i} & \boldsymbol{\Sigma}_{(i+1)} \end{pmatrix} \begin{pmatrix} 1 & \boldsymbol{\gamma}_{(i)}^\top \\ \boldsymbol{0}_{p-i} & \boldsymbol{I}_{p-i} \end{pmatrix}. \tag{3.6}$$

Similarly, for $i = 1, \ldots, \nu$, let $\boldsymbol{T}_{(i)}$ be submatrices obtained by removing the first $(i-1)$ rows and columns of $\boldsymbol{T} = (t_{i,j}) \in \mathbb{L}_{p,\nu}^{(+)}$. For $i = 1, \ldots, \nu-1$, partition $\boldsymbol{T}_{(i)}$ into four blocks as

$$\boldsymbol{T}_{(i)} = \begin{pmatrix} t_{i,i} & \boldsymbol{0}_{p-i}^\top \\ \boldsymbol{t}_{(i)} & \boldsymbol{T}_{(i+1)} \end{pmatrix} \in \mathbb{L}_{p-i+1,\nu-i+1}^{(+)},$$

where $\boldsymbol{t}_{(i)} = (t_{i+1,i}, \ldots, t_{p,i})^\top$. Note that for $i = 1, \ldots, \nu-1$

$$\boldsymbol{T}_{(i)}\boldsymbol{T}_{(i)}^\top = \begin{pmatrix} 1 & \boldsymbol{0}_{p-i}^\top \\ t_{i,i}^{-1}\boldsymbol{t}_{(i)} & \boldsymbol{I}_{p-i} \end{pmatrix} \begin{pmatrix} t_{i,i}^2 & \boldsymbol{0}_{p-i}^\top \\ \boldsymbol{0}_{p-i} & \boldsymbol{T}_{(i+1)}\boldsymbol{T}_{(i+1)}^\top \end{pmatrix} \begin{pmatrix} 1 & t_{i,i}^{-1}\boldsymbol{t}_{(i)}^\top \\ \boldsymbol{0}_{p-i} & \boldsymbol{I}_{p-i} \end{pmatrix} \tag{3.7}$$

and

$$\boldsymbol{T}_{(\nu)} = (t_{\nu,\nu}, t_{\nu+1,\nu}, \dots, t_{p,\nu})^\top = \begin{cases} t_{p,p} & \text{for } n \geq p \ (\nu = p), \\ (t_{n,n}, t_{n+1,n}, \dots, t_{p,n})^\top & \text{for } p > n \ (\nu = n). \end{cases}$$

In the $p > n$ case, define additionally $\boldsymbol{T}_{(n)} = (t_{n,n}, \boldsymbol{t}_{(n)}^\top)^\top$ with $\boldsymbol{t}_{(n)} = (t_{n+1,n}, \dots, t_{p,n})^\top$. Then we have the following proposition.

Proposition 3.10 *The columns of $\boldsymbol{T}$ are mutually independent and*

$$\begin{cases} t_{i,i}^2 \sim \sigma_i^2 \chi_{n-i+1}^2 & \text{for } i = 1, \dots, \nu, \\ \boldsymbol{t}_{(i)} | t_{i,i} \sim N_{p-i}(t_{i,i}\boldsymbol{\gamma}_{(i)}, \boldsymbol{\Sigma}_{(i+1)}) & \text{for } i = 1, \dots, n \wedge (p-1). \end{cases} \tag{3.8}$$

Proof From Proposition 3.9, it is immediately seen that the columns of $\boldsymbol{T}$ are mutually independent. Using (3.6) and (3.7) gives

$$\operatorname{tr} \boldsymbol{\Sigma}_{(i)}^{-1} \boldsymbol{T}_{(i)} \boldsymbol{T}_{(i)}^\top = t_{i,i}^2/\sigma_i^2 + (\boldsymbol{t}_{(i)} - t_{i,i}\boldsymbol{\gamma}_{(i)})^\top \boldsymbol{\Sigma}_{(i+1)}^{-1} (\boldsymbol{t}_{(i)} - t_{i,i}\boldsymbol{\gamma}_{(i)}) + \operatorname{tr} \boldsymbol{\Sigma}_{(i+1)}^{-1} \boldsymbol{T}_{(i+1)} \boldsymbol{T}_{(i+1)}^\top,$$

so that

$$\begin{aligned} \operatorname{tr} \boldsymbol{\Sigma}^{-1} \boldsymbol{T}\boldsymbol{T}^\top &= t_{1,1}^2/\sigma_1^2 + (\boldsymbol{t}_{(1)} - t_{1,1}\boldsymbol{\gamma}_{(1)})^\top \boldsymbol{\Sigma}_{(2)}^{-1} (\boldsymbol{t}_{(1)} - t_{1,1}\boldsymbol{\gamma}_{(1)}) + \operatorname{tr} \boldsymbol{\Sigma}_{(2)}^{-1} \boldsymbol{T}_{(2)} \boldsymbol{T}_{(2)}^\top \\ &= \sum_{i=1}^{2} \frac{t_{i,i}^2}{\sigma_i^2} + \sum_{i=1}^{2} (\boldsymbol{t}_{(i)} - t_{i,i}\boldsymbol{\gamma}_{(i)})^\top \boldsymbol{\Sigma}_{(i+1)}^{-1} (\boldsymbol{t}_{(i)} - t_{i,i}\boldsymbol{\gamma}_{(i)}) + \operatorname{tr} \boldsymbol{\Sigma}_{(3)}^{-1} \boldsymbol{T}_{(3)} \boldsymbol{T}_{(3)}^\top \\ &= \cdots \\ &= \sum_{i=1}^{\nu} \frac{t_{i,i}^2}{\sigma_i^2} + \sum_{i=1}^{n\wedge(p-1)} (\boldsymbol{t}_{(i)} - t_{i,i}\boldsymbol{\gamma}_{(i)})^\top \boldsymbol{\Sigma}_{(i+1)}^{-1} (\boldsymbol{t}_{(i)} - t_{i,i}\boldsymbol{\gamma}_{(i)}). \end{aligned}$$

Also, for $i = 1, \dots, p-1$,

$$|\boldsymbol{\Sigma}| = |\boldsymbol{\Sigma}_{(2)}|\sigma_1^2 = |\boldsymbol{\Sigma}_{(3)}| \prod_{j=1}^{2} \sigma_j^2 = \cdots = |\boldsymbol{\Sigma}_{(i+1)}| \prod_{j=1}^{i} \sigma_j^2,$$

yielding

$$|\boldsymbol{\Sigma}|^{n/2} = \left(\prod_{i=1}^{n\wedge(p-1)} |\boldsymbol{\Sigma}_{(i+1)}|^{1/2} \right) \left(\prod_{i=1}^{\nu} (\sigma_i^2)^{(n-i+1)/2} \right).$$

It turns out from Proposition 3.1 that

$$\frac{2^\nu \pi^{n\nu/2}}{(2\pi)^{np/2} \Gamma_\nu(n/2)} = \left(\prod_{i=1}^{n\wedge(p-1)} \frac{1}{(2\pi)^{(p-i)/2}} \right) \left(\prod_{i=1}^{\nu} \frac{2}{2^{(n-i+1)/2} \Gamma((n-i+1)/2)} \right),$$

so that the p.d.f. of $\boldsymbol{T}$, given in Proposition 3.9, can be rewritten as

$$\prod_{i=1}^{n\wedge(p-1)} \frac{1}{(2\pi)^{(p-i)/2}|\boldsymbol{\Sigma}_{(i+1)}|^{1/2}} \exp\left(-\frac{1}{2}(\boldsymbol{t}_{(i)} - t_{i,i}\boldsymbol{\gamma}_{(i)})^\top \boldsymbol{\Sigma}_{(i+1)}^{-1}(\boldsymbol{t}_{(i)} - t_{i,i}\boldsymbol{\gamma}_{(i)})\right)$$
$$\times \prod_{i=1}^{\nu} \frac{2}{2^{(n-i+1)/2}\Gamma((n-i+1)/2)}(\sigma_i^2)^{-(n-i+1)/2} t_{i,i}^{n-i} \exp\left(-\frac{t_{i,i}^2}{2\sigma_i^2}\right).$$

Thus, for $i = 1, \ldots, n \wedge (p-1)$, $\boldsymbol{t}_{(i)}|t_{i,i} \sim \mathcal{N}_{p-i}(t_{i,i}\boldsymbol{\gamma}_{(i)}, \boldsymbol{\Sigma}_{(i+1)})$. Finally, making the change of variables $y_i = t_{i,i}^2$ for $i = 1, \ldots, \nu$ gives $y_i \sim \sigma_i^2 \chi_{n-i+1}^2$. □

The distributional decomposition (3.8) will be used in Sect. 7.6 for estimation of a covariance matrix.

Proposition 3.10 immediately provides the following corollary.

Corollary 3.2 *Let* $\boldsymbol{X} \sim \mathcal{N}_{n\times p}(\boldsymbol{0}_{n\times p}, \boldsymbol{I}_n \otimes \boldsymbol{I}_p)$. *Denote by* $\boldsymbol{X}^\top\boldsymbol{X} = \boldsymbol{T}\boldsymbol{T}^\top$ *the Cholesky decomposition of* $\boldsymbol{X}^\top\boldsymbol{X}$, *where* $\boldsymbol{T} = (t_{i,j}) \in \mathbb{L}_{p,\nu}^{(+)}$ *with* $\nu = n \wedge p$. *Then all the nonzero elements of* $\boldsymbol{T}$ *are mutually independent and distributed as*

$$\begin{cases} t_{i,i}^2 \sim \chi_{n-i+1}^2 & \text{for } i = 1, \ldots, \nu, \\ t_{i,j} \sim \mathcal{N}(0, 1) & \text{for } 2 \le i \le p \text{ and } 1 \le j \le n \wedge (i-1). \end{cases}$$

References

J.A. Díaz-García, R. Gutierrez-Jáimez, K.V. Mardia, Wishart and pseudo-Wishart distributions and some applications to shape theory. J. Multivar. Anal. **63**, 73–87 (1997)

A.K. Gupta, D.K. Nagar, *Matrix Variate Distributions* (Chapman & Hall/CRC, New York, 1999)

A.M. Mathai, *Jacobian of Matrix Transformations and Functions of Matrix Argument* (World Scientific, Singapore, 1997)

R.J. Muirhead, *Aspects of Multivariate Statistical Theory* (Wiley, New York, 1982)

M.S. Srivastava, C.G. Khatri, *An Introduction to Multivariate Statistics* (North Holland, New York, 1979)

H. Uhlig, On singular Wishart and singular multivariate Beta distributions. Ann. Stat. **22**, 395–405 (1994)

J. Wishart, The generalised product moment distribution in samples from a normal multivariate population. Biometrika **20**, 32–52 (1928)

Chapter 4
Multivariate Linear Model and Group Invariance

Multivariate linear model is a multivariate generalization for the dimension of response variable in traditional multiple linear regression model. This chapter provides some fundamental properties in terms of the multivariate linear model and the corresponding canonical form. The group invariance is also explained for shrinkage estimation in the multivariate linear model.

4.1 Multivariate Linear Model

The sample size is denoted by N. For $i = 1, \dots, N$, let $\boldsymbol{y}_i$ be a p-dimensional column vector of response variables and let

$$\boldsymbol{y}_i = \boldsymbol{B}^\top \boldsymbol{x}_i + \boldsymbol{\varepsilon}_i,$$

where $\boldsymbol{x}_i \in \mathbb{R}^m$ is a column vector of known explanatory variables ($m \le N$), $\boldsymbol{B} \in \mathbb{R}^{m\times p}$ is a matrix of unknown parameters and $\boldsymbol{\varepsilon}_i \in \mathbb{R}^p$ is a random vector. Define $\boldsymbol{Y} = (\boldsymbol{y}_1, \dots, \boldsymbol{y}_N)^\top \in \mathbb{R}^{N\times p}$, $\boldsymbol{X} = (\boldsymbol{x}_1, \dots, \boldsymbol{x}_N)^\top \in \mathbb{R}^{N\times m}$ and $\boldsymbol{E} = (\boldsymbol{\varepsilon}_1, \dots, \boldsymbol{\varepsilon}_N)^\top \in \mathbb{R}^{N\times p}$. Then we obtain

$$\boldsymbol{Y} = \boldsymbol{X}\boldsymbol{B} + \boldsymbol{E}. \tag{4.1}$$

Assume that for $i = 1, \dots, N$ the $\boldsymbol{\varepsilon}_i$'s are independently distributed as $\mathcal{N}_p(\boldsymbol{0}_p, \boldsymbol{\Sigma})$, namely, the error matrix $\boldsymbol{E}$ follows $\mathcal{N}_{N\times p}(\boldsymbol{0}_{N\times p}, \boldsymbol{I}_N \otimes \boldsymbol{\Sigma})$, where $\boldsymbol{\Sigma} \in \mathbb{S}_p^{(+)}$ is unknown. In addition, $\boldsymbol{X}$ is assumed to be of full column rank.

In the literature, model (4.1) is called the multivariate linear model or multivariate linear regression model, and the parameter matrix $\boldsymbol{B}$ is called the regression coefficient matrix or simply the regression matrix. The multivariate linear model (4.1) is closely relevant to various models from simple to complex, such as a simple

H. Tsukuma and T. Kubokawa, *Shrinkage Estimation for Mean and Covariance Matrices*, JSS Research Series in Statistics, https://doi.org/10.1007/978-981-15-1596-5_4

mean-variance model, the multivariate analysis of variance (MANOVA) model and the growth curve model.

We now consider estimation of $\boldsymbol{B}$. There are many procedures for estimation of $\boldsymbol{B}$, and we here introduce the least squares method that is one of the most well-known procedures. Let

$$g(\boldsymbol{B}) = \sum_{i=1}^{N} \|\boldsymbol{y}_i - \boldsymbol{B}^\top \boldsymbol{x}_i\|^2,$$

where $\|\cdot\|$ denotes the usual Euclidean norm. Then the least squares method is the minimization of $g(\boldsymbol{B})$ subject to $\boldsymbol{B}$. Noting that

$$\boldsymbol{Y}^\top \boldsymbol{Y} = \sum_{i=1}^{N} \boldsymbol{y}_i \boldsymbol{y}_i^\top, \quad \boldsymbol{X}^\top \boldsymbol{Y} = \sum_{i=1}^{N} \boldsymbol{x}_i \boldsymbol{y}_i^\top, \quad \boldsymbol{X}^\top \boldsymbol{X} = \sum_{i=1}^{N} \boldsymbol{x}_i \boldsymbol{x}_i^\top,$$

we observe that

$$\begin{aligned} g(\boldsymbol{B}) &= \sum_{i=1}^{N} \operatorname{tr}(\boldsymbol{y}_i - \boldsymbol{B}^\top \boldsymbol{x}_i)(\boldsymbol{y}_i - \boldsymbol{B}^\top \boldsymbol{x}_i)^\top \\ &= \operatorname{tr}(\boldsymbol{Y}^\top \boldsymbol{Y} - \boldsymbol{B}^\top \boldsymbol{X}^\top \boldsymbol{Y} - \boldsymbol{Y}^\top \boldsymbol{X} \boldsymbol{B} + \boldsymbol{B}^\top \boldsymbol{X}^\top \boldsymbol{X} \boldsymbol{B}). \end{aligned}$$

Recall that $\boldsymbol{X}$ is of full column rank, and thus $\boldsymbol{X}^\top \boldsymbol{X}$ is nonsingular. Completing the square with respect to $\boldsymbol{B}$ gives

$$g(\boldsymbol{B}) = \operatorname{tr}(\boldsymbol{B} - \widehat{\boldsymbol{B}})^\top \boldsymbol{X}^\top \boldsymbol{X}(\boldsymbol{B} - \widehat{\boldsymbol{B}}) + \operatorname{tr}(\boldsymbol{Y}^\top \boldsymbol{Y} - \widehat{\boldsymbol{B}}^\top \boldsymbol{X}^\top \boldsymbol{X} \widehat{\boldsymbol{B}}),$$

where

$$\widehat{\boldsymbol{B}} = (\boldsymbol{X}^\top \boldsymbol{X})^{-1} \boldsymbol{X}^\top \boldsymbol{Y}.$$

Clearly $g(\boldsymbol{B})$ is minimized at $\boldsymbol{B} = \widehat{\boldsymbol{B}}$. The resulting $\widehat{\boldsymbol{B}}$ is called the least squares (LS) estimator of $\boldsymbol{B}$. Since $\boldsymbol{E} \sim \mathcal{N}_{N\times p}(\boldsymbol{0}_{N\times p}, \boldsymbol{I}_N \otimes \boldsymbol{\Sigma})$ in (4.1), namely, $\boldsymbol{Y} \sim \mathcal{N}_{N\times p}(\boldsymbol{X}\boldsymbol{B}, \boldsymbol{I}_N \otimes \boldsymbol{\Sigma})$, the likelihood without a normalizing constant can be written as

$$|\boldsymbol{\Sigma}|^{-N/2} \exp\Big[-\frac{1}{2} \operatorname{tr} \boldsymbol{\Sigma}^{-1} \{(\boldsymbol{B} - \widehat{\boldsymbol{B}})^\top \boldsymbol{X}^\top \boldsymbol{X}(\boldsymbol{B} - \widehat{\boldsymbol{B}}) + (\boldsymbol{Y}^\top \boldsymbol{Y} - \widehat{\boldsymbol{B}}^\top \boldsymbol{X}^\top \boldsymbol{X} \widehat{\boldsymbol{B}})\}\Big].$$

Thus the LS estimator $\widehat{\boldsymbol{B}}$ is the maximum likelihood estimator as well. Also, using Proposition 3.5 leads to

$$\widehat{\boldsymbol{B}} \sim \mathcal{N}_{m\times p}(\boldsymbol{B}, (\boldsymbol{X}^\top \boldsymbol{X})^{-1} \otimes \boldsymbol{\Sigma}),$$

implying that $\widehat{\boldsymbol{B}}$ is an unbiased estimator of $\boldsymbol{B}$.

Next we find a reasonable estimator for the covariance matrix $\boldsymbol{\Sigma}$ of random error terms $\boldsymbol{\varepsilon}_i$'s in the multivariate linear model (4.1). In traditional multiple linear regression model, a residual sum of squares is often used to estimate an error variance, which can be extended to estimating the error covariance $\boldsymbol{\Sigma}$.

Let

$$\boldsymbol{S} = \sum_{i=1}^{N}(\boldsymbol{y}_i - \widehat{\boldsymbol{B}}^\top \boldsymbol{x}_i)(\boldsymbol{y}_i - \widehat{\boldsymbol{B}}^\top \boldsymbol{x}_i)^\top,$$

which is called the residual sum of squares matrix. It turns out that

$$\begin{aligned}\sum_{i=1}^{N}(\boldsymbol{y}_i - \widehat{\boldsymbol{B}}^\top \boldsymbol{x}_i)(\boldsymbol{y}_i - \widehat{\boldsymbol{B}}^\top \boldsymbol{x}_i)^\top &= \boldsymbol{Y}^\top \boldsymbol{Y} - \widehat{\boldsymbol{B}}^\top \boldsymbol{X}^\top \boldsymbol{Y} - \boldsymbol{Y}^\top \boldsymbol{X}\widehat{\boldsymbol{B}} + \widehat{\boldsymbol{B}}^\top \boldsymbol{X}^\top \boldsymbol{X}\widehat{\boldsymbol{B}} \\ &= \boldsymbol{Y}^\top \{\boldsymbol{I}_N - \boldsymbol{X}(\boldsymbol{X}^\top \boldsymbol{X})^{-1}\boldsymbol{X}^\top\}\boldsymbol{Y},\end{aligned}$$

so that

$$\boldsymbol{S} = \boldsymbol{Y}^\top(\boldsymbol{I}_N - \boldsymbol{P}_X)\boldsymbol{Y},$$

where $\boldsymbol{P}_X = \boldsymbol{X}(\boldsymbol{X}^\top \boldsymbol{X})^{-1}\boldsymbol{X}^\top$. Here, $\boldsymbol{P}_X$ is the orthogonal projection matrix onto the subspace spanned by columns of $\boldsymbol{X}$. Now, we write the QR decomposition of $\boldsymbol{X}$ as $\boldsymbol{X} = \boldsymbol{Q}_1 \boldsymbol{L}^\top$, where $\boldsymbol{Q}_1 \in \mathbb{V}_{N,m}$ and $\boldsymbol{L} \in \mathbb{L}_m^{(+)}$. There exists $\boldsymbol{Q}_2 \in \mathbb{V}_{N,n}$ for $n = N - m$ such that $(\boldsymbol{Q}_1, \boldsymbol{Q}_2) \in \mathbb{O}_N$, namely, the set of N columns of an $N \times N$ matrix $(\boldsymbol{Q}_1, \boldsymbol{Q}_2)$ forms an orthonormal basis of $\mathbb{R}^N$. Then

$$P_X = \boldsymbol{Q}_1 \boldsymbol{L}^\top (\boldsymbol{L}\boldsymbol{Q}_1^\top \boldsymbol{Q}_1 \boldsymbol{L}^\top)^{-1} \boldsymbol{L}\boldsymbol{Q}_1^\top = \boldsymbol{Q}_1 \boldsymbol{Q}_1^\top$$

and $\boldsymbol{I}_N - \boldsymbol{P}_X = \boldsymbol{I}_N - \boldsymbol{Q}_1 \boldsymbol{Q}_1^\top = \boldsymbol{Q}_2 \boldsymbol{Q}_2^\top$. Since $\boldsymbol{Q}_2^\top \boldsymbol{X}\boldsymbol{B} = \boldsymbol{Q}_2^\top \boldsymbol{Q}_1 \boldsymbol{L}^\top \boldsymbol{B} = \boldsymbol{0}_{n\times p}$, using Proposition 3.5 gives $\boldsymbol{Q}_2^\top \boldsymbol{Y} \sim N_{n\times p}(\boldsymbol{0}_{n\times p}, \boldsymbol{I}_n \otimes \boldsymbol{\Sigma})$. From Definition 3.3,

$$\boldsymbol{S} = \boldsymbol{Y}^\top \boldsymbol{Q}_2 \boldsymbol{Q}_2^\top \boldsymbol{Y} \sim \mathcal{W}_p^\nu(n, \boldsymbol{\Sigma})$$

with $\nu = n \wedge p$. Hence, by Proposition 3.8,

$$\widehat{\boldsymbol{\Sigma}}^{UB} = \frac{1}{n}\boldsymbol{S}, \quad n = N - m,$$

is unbiased for $\boldsymbol{\Sigma}$.

The unbiased estimator $\widehat{\boldsymbol{\Sigma}}^{UB}$ is reasonable, but not the maximum likelihood estimator of $\boldsymbol{\Sigma}$. Note that $(\widehat{\boldsymbol{B}}, \widehat{\boldsymbol{\Sigma}}^{UB})$, or $(\widehat{\boldsymbol{B}}, \boldsymbol{S})$, is a sufficient statistic for $(\boldsymbol{B}, \boldsymbol{\Sigma})$. See Muirhead (1982, Theorem 10.1.1) or Anderson (2003, Corollary 8.2.1).

4.2 A Canonical Form

Let $\boldsymbol{Q} = (\boldsymbol{Q}_1, \boldsymbol{Q}_2) \in \mathbb{O}_N$, where $\boldsymbol{Q}_1$ and $\boldsymbol{Q}_2$ are defined as in the previous section. Then

$$\boldsymbol{Q}^\top \boldsymbol{X} = \begin{pmatrix} \boldsymbol{Q}_1^\top \boldsymbol{X} \\ \boldsymbol{Q}_2^\top \boldsymbol{X} \end{pmatrix} = \begin{pmatrix} \boldsymbol{L}^\top \\ \boldsymbol{0}_{n\times m} \end{pmatrix}$$

for $n = N - m$. Let $\boldsymbol{\Theta} = (\boldsymbol{\theta}_1, \dots, \boldsymbol{\theta}_m)^\top = \boldsymbol{L}^\top \boldsymbol{B} \in \mathbb{R}^{m\times p}$. Define

$$\begin{pmatrix} \boldsymbol{Z} \\ \boldsymbol{U} \end{pmatrix} = \boldsymbol{Q}^\top \boldsymbol{Y} = \begin{pmatrix} \boldsymbol{Q}_1^\top \boldsymbol{Y} \\ \boldsymbol{Q}_2^\top \boldsymbol{Y} \end{pmatrix},$$

where $\boldsymbol{Z} = (\boldsymbol{z}_1, \dots, \boldsymbol{z}_m)^\top \in \mathbb{R}^{m\times p}$ and $\boldsymbol{U} = (\boldsymbol{u}_1, \dots, \boldsymbol{u}_n)^\top \in \mathbb{R}^{n\times p}$.

Recall that $\boldsymbol{Y} \sim \mathcal{N}_{N\times p}(\boldsymbol{XB}, \boldsymbol{I}_N \otimes \boldsymbol{\Sigma})$, so that by Proposition 3.5

$$\begin{pmatrix} \boldsymbol{Z} \\ \boldsymbol{U} \end{pmatrix} \sim \mathcal{N}_{N\times p}\left(\begin{pmatrix} \boldsymbol{\Theta} \\ \boldsymbol{0}_{n\times p} \end{pmatrix}, \boldsymbol{I}_N \otimes \boldsymbol{\Sigma} \right).$$

Hence from Proposition 3.6, $\boldsymbol{Z}$ and $\boldsymbol{U}$ are independently distributed as

$$\boldsymbol{Z} \sim \mathcal{N}_{m\times p}(\boldsymbol{\Theta}, \boldsymbol{I}_m \otimes \boldsymbol{\Sigma}), \qquad \boldsymbol{U} \sim \mathcal{N}_{n\times p}(\boldsymbol{0}_{n\times p}, \boldsymbol{I}_n \otimes \boldsymbol{\Sigma}), \tag{4.2}$$

which is a canonical form of the multivariate linear model (4.1). The canonical form (4.2) is equivalent to

$$\begin{aligned} \boldsymbol{z}_i &\sim \mathcal{N}_p(\boldsymbol{\theta}_i, \boldsymbol{\Sigma}), \quad i = 1, \dots, m, \\ \boldsymbol{u}_j &\sim \mathcal{N}_p(\boldsymbol{0}_p, \boldsymbol{\Sigma}), \quad j = 1, \dots, n, \end{aligned}$$

where all of the $\boldsymbol{z}_i$'s and $\boldsymbol{u}_j$'s are mutually independent.

The QR decomposition of $\boldsymbol{X}$ is denoted by $\boldsymbol{X} = \boldsymbol{Q}_1 \boldsymbol{L}^\top$, yielding

$$\widehat{\boldsymbol{B}} = (\boldsymbol{X}^\top \boldsymbol{X})^{-1} \boldsymbol{X}^\top \boldsymbol{Y} = (\boldsymbol{L}\boldsymbol{Q}_1^\top \boldsymbol{Q}_1 \boldsymbol{L}^\top)^{-1} \boldsymbol{L}\boldsymbol{Q}_1^\top \boldsymbol{Y} = (\boldsymbol{L}^\top)^{-1} \boldsymbol{Z},$$

namely, $\boldsymbol{Z} = \boldsymbol{L}^\top \widehat{\boldsymbol{B}}$. Here,

$$\boldsymbol{S} = \boldsymbol{U}^\top \boldsymbol{U} = \sum_{i=1}^n \boldsymbol{u}_i \boldsymbol{u}_i^\top$$

is also called the Wishart matrix, which follows $\mathcal{W}_p^\nu(n, \boldsymbol{\Sigma})$ with $\nu = n \wedge p$. Thus $\widehat{\boldsymbol{B}}$ and $\boldsymbol{S}$ are, respectively, made from $\boldsymbol{Z}$ and $\boldsymbol{U}$, and are mutually independent. From (4.2), $(\boldsymbol{Z}, \boldsymbol{U})$ is a sufficient statistic of $(\boldsymbol{\Theta}, \boldsymbol{\Sigma})$.

In this book, $\boldsymbol{\Theta}$ and $\boldsymbol{\Sigma}$ are hereinafter called the mean and the covariance matrices, respectively, and the estimation problem for $\boldsymbol{\Theta}$ and $\boldsymbol{\Sigma}$ will be treated in the canonical form (4.2).

4.3 Group Invariance

If an estimation problem is invariant under a transformation such as translation, scaling and rotation, it seems reasonable to require all decision rules, namely, all possible estimators are invariant under the transformation. In this section, we briefly provide the definition of group invariance, or simply called invariance, and simple examples in the canonical form (4.2) of the multivariate linear model (4.1).

Let P_θ be a probability distribution on a sample space $\mathcal{X}$ parameterized by θ. A statistical model $\mathcal{M}$ is defined by $\mathcal{M} = \{P_\theta : \theta \in \mathcal{P}\}$, namely, it is a family of probability distributions P_θ, where $\mathcal{P}$ is a parameter space. Let x be an observed random variable having P_θ and suppose θ is estimated by using x. Denote by $\hat{\theta} = \hat{\theta}(x)$ an estimator of θ based on x, and by $\mathcal{D}$ a decision space consisting of all possible estimators $\hat{\theta}$. A distance between θ and its estimator $\hat{\theta}$ is measured by a loss function $L(\hat{\theta}, \theta)$.

Let $\mathbb{G}$ be a transformation group which acts on $\mathcal{X}$. For any $g \in \mathbb{G}$, the group action on $x \in \mathcal{X}$ is written as gx. A statistical model $\mathcal{M}$ is said to be invariant under $\mathbb{G}$ if, for any $g \in \mathbb{G}$ and $\theta \in \mathcal{P}$, there exists a unique $\bar{g}\theta \in \mathcal{P}$ such that a distribution of gx is $P_{\bar{g}\theta} \in \mathcal{M}$. For an invariant statistical model $\mathcal{M}$ under $\mathbb{G}$, all of the $\bar{g}$'s form a group of transformations from $\mathcal{P}$ into itself and it is called the group induced by $\mathbb{G}$. When a statistical model $\mathcal{M}$ is invariant under $\mathbb{G}$, a loss function $L(\hat{\theta}, \theta)$ is said to be invariant under $\mathbb{G}$ if, for any $g \in \mathbb{G}$ and $\hat{\theta} \in \mathcal{D}$, there exists an estimator $\tilde{g}\hat{\theta}$ such that $L(\tilde{g}\hat{\theta}, \bar{g}\theta) = L(\hat{\theta}, \theta)$ for any $\theta \in \mathcal{P}$. Note that all of the $\tilde{g}$'s also form a group of transformations from $\mathcal{D}$ into itself. An estimator $\hat{\theta}(x)$ is said to be invariant under $\mathbb{G}$ if $\hat{\theta}(gx) = \tilde{g}\hat{\theta}(x)$ for any $g \in \mathbb{G}$ and $x \in \mathcal{X}$. An estimation problem is said to be invariant under $\mathbb{G}$ if the model $\mathcal{M}$ and the loss function L are invariant under $\mathbb{G}$.

Now, simple examples of invariance are given in terms of the canonical form (4.2) of the multivariate linear model (4.1), which is rewritten as

$$\boldsymbol{X} \sim \mathcal{N}_{m\times p}(\boldsymbol{\Theta}, \boldsymbol{I}_m \otimes \boldsymbol{\Sigma}), \qquad \boldsymbol{Y} \sim \mathcal{N}_{n\times p}(\boldsymbol{0}_{n\times p}, \boldsymbol{I}_n \otimes \boldsymbol{\Sigma}), \tag{4.3}$$

where $\boldsymbol{\Theta} \in \mathbb{R}^{m\times p}$ and $\boldsymbol{\Sigma} \in \mathbb{S}_p^{(+)}$. Consider the problem of estimating the mean matrix $\boldsymbol{\Theta}$ relative to the quadratic loss $L_Q(\widehat{\boldsymbol{\Theta}}, \theta) = \operatorname{tr}(\widehat{\boldsymbol{\Theta}} - \boldsymbol{\Theta})\boldsymbol{\Sigma}^{-1}(\widehat{\boldsymbol{\Theta}} - \boldsymbol{\Theta})^\top$, where $\widehat{\boldsymbol{\Theta}} = \widehat{\boldsymbol{\Theta}}(x)$ with $x = (\boldsymbol{X}, \boldsymbol{Y})$ and $\theta = (\boldsymbol{\Theta}, \boldsymbol{\Sigma})$.

In the model (4.3), the sample and the parameter spaces are, respectively, $\mathcal{X} = \mathbb{R}^{m\times p} \times \mathbb{R}^{n\times p}$ and $\mathcal{P} = \mathbb{R}^{m\times p} \times \mathbb{S}_p^{(+)}$. The decision space is denoted by $\mathcal{D} = \{\widehat{\boldsymbol{\Theta}}(x) \in \mathbb{R}^{m\times p} : x \in \mathcal{X}\}$. We define the transformation group $\mathbb{G}$ as

$$\mathbb{G} = \{(\boldsymbol{O}, \boldsymbol{U}) : \ \boldsymbol{O} \in \mathbb{O}_m \text{ and } \boldsymbol{U} \in \mathbb{U}_p\}$$

with operation $g_1 g_2 = (\boldsymbol{O}_1\boldsymbol{O}_2, \boldsymbol{U}_2\boldsymbol{U}_1)$ for any $g_1 = (\boldsymbol{O}_1, \boldsymbol{U}_1),\ g_2 = (\boldsymbol{O}_2, \boldsymbol{U}_2) \in \mathbb{G}$. The group action of $g = (\boldsymbol{O}, \boldsymbol{U}) \in \mathbb{G}$ on $x \in \mathcal{X}$ and the induced group actions $\bar{g}$ on $\theta \in \mathcal{P}$ and $\tilde{g}$ on $\widehat{\boldsymbol{\Theta}} \in \mathcal{D}$ are given, respectively, by scale transformations

$$
\begin{aligned}
x &\to gx = (\boldsymbol{O}\boldsymbol{X}\boldsymbol{U}, \boldsymbol{Y}\boldsymbol{U}), \\
\theta &\to \tilde{g}\theta = (\boldsymbol{O}\boldsymbol{\Theta}\boldsymbol{U}, \boldsymbol{U}^\top \boldsymbol{\Sigma}\boldsymbol{U}), \\
\widehat{\boldsymbol{\Theta}} &\to \tilde{g}\widehat{\boldsymbol{\Theta}} = \boldsymbol{O}\widehat{\boldsymbol{\Theta}}\boldsymbol{U}.
\end{aligned}
\tag{4.4}
$$

From Proposition 3.5, it is easy to see that the model (4.3) is invariant under $\mathbb{G}$. Also, the invariance of the L_Q-loss can be verified because

$$
\begin{aligned}
L_Q(\tilde{g}\widehat{\boldsymbol{\Theta}}, \tilde{g}\theta) &= \operatorname{tr}(\boldsymbol{O}\widehat{\boldsymbol{\Theta}}\boldsymbol{U} - \boldsymbol{O}\boldsymbol{\Theta}\boldsymbol{U})(\boldsymbol{U}^\top\boldsymbol{\Sigma}\boldsymbol{U})^{-1}(\boldsymbol{O}\widehat{\boldsymbol{\Theta}}\boldsymbol{U} - \boldsymbol{O}\boldsymbol{\Theta}\boldsymbol{U})^\top \\
&= \operatorname{tr}(\widehat{\boldsymbol{\Theta}} - \boldsymbol{\Theta})\boldsymbol{\Sigma}^{-1}(\widehat{\boldsymbol{\Theta}} - \boldsymbol{\Theta})^\top = L_Q(\widehat{\boldsymbol{\Theta}}, \theta).
\end{aligned}
$$

Thus the estimation problem of $\boldsymbol{\Theta}$ in (4.3) relative to the L_Q-loss is invariant under $\mathbb{G}$.

Let $\boldsymbol{S} = \boldsymbol{Y}^\top\boldsymbol{Y}$. For $n \geq p$, let an estimator of $\boldsymbol{\Theta}$ be

$$
\widehat{\boldsymbol{\Theta}} = \widehat{\boldsymbol{\Theta}}(x) = \begin{cases} \boldsymbol{X}(\boldsymbol{I}_p - c_1(\boldsymbol{X}^\top\boldsymbol{X})^{-1}\boldsymbol{S}) & \text{for } m > p, \\ (\boldsymbol{I}_m - c_2(\boldsymbol{X}\boldsymbol{S}^{-1}\boldsymbol{X}^\top)^{-1})\boldsymbol{X} & \text{for } p \geq m, \end{cases}
$$

where c_1 and c_2 are positive constants. When $n \geq p$, $\boldsymbol{S}$ belongs to $\mathbb{S}_p^{(+)}$ with probability one. Here $\widehat{\boldsymbol{\Theta}}$ is invariant under $\mathbb{G}$. Indeed, for $m > p$,

$$
\begin{aligned}
\widehat{\boldsymbol{\Theta}}(gx) &= \boldsymbol{O}\boldsymbol{X}\boldsymbol{U}[\boldsymbol{I}_p - c_1\{(\boldsymbol{O}\boldsymbol{X}\boldsymbol{U})^\top\boldsymbol{O}\boldsymbol{X}\boldsymbol{U}\}^{-1}\boldsymbol{U}^\top\boldsymbol{S}\boldsymbol{U}] \\
&= \boldsymbol{O}\boldsymbol{X}\{\boldsymbol{I}_p - c_1(\boldsymbol{X}^\top\boldsymbol{X})^{-1}\boldsymbol{S}\}\boldsymbol{U} \\
&= \boldsymbol{O}\widehat{\boldsymbol{\Theta}}(x)\boldsymbol{U} = \tilde{g}\widehat{\boldsymbol{\Theta}}(x),
\end{aligned}
$$

and for $p \geq m$

$$
\begin{aligned}
\widehat{\boldsymbol{\Theta}}(gx) &= [\boldsymbol{I}_m - c_2\{\boldsymbol{O}\boldsymbol{X}\boldsymbol{U}(\boldsymbol{U}^\top\boldsymbol{S}\boldsymbol{U})^{-1}(\boldsymbol{O}\boldsymbol{X}\boldsymbol{U})^\top\}^{-1}]\boldsymbol{O}\boldsymbol{X}\boldsymbol{U} \\
&= \boldsymbol{O}\{\boldsymbol{I}_m - c_2(\boldsymbol{X}\boldsymbol{S}^{-1}\boldsymbol{X}^\top)^{-1}\}\boldsymbol{X}\boldsymbol{U} \\
&= \boldsymbol{O}\widehat{\boldsymbol{\Theta}}(x)\boldsymbol{U} = \tilde{g}\widehat{\boldsymbol{\Theta}}(x).
\end{aligned}
$$

On the other hand, for example, an estimator $\widehat{\boldsymbol{\Theta}}_0 = \boldsymbol{X} - \boldsymbol{X}/\operatorname{tr}\boldsymbol{X}\boldsymbol{X}^\top$ is not invariant under $\mathbb{G}$. Further, a quadratic-type loss $L_F(\widehat{\boldsymbol{\Theta}}, \theta) = \operatorname{tr}(\widehat{\boldsymbol{\Theta}} - \boldsymbol{\Theta})(\widehat{\boldsymbol{\Theta}} - \boldsymbol{\Theta})^\top$ is not invariant under $\mathbb{G}$ since

$$
\begin{aligned}
L_F(\tilde{g}\widehat{\boldsymbol{\Theta}}, \tilde{g}\theta) &= \operatorname{tr}(\boldsymbol{O}\widehat{\boldsymbol{\Theta}}\boldsymbol{U} - \boldsymbol{O}\boldsymbol{\Theta}\boldsymbol{U})(\boldsymbol{O}\widehat{\boldsymbol{\Theta}}\boldsymbol{U} - \boldsymbol{O}\boldsymbol{\Theta}\boldsymbol{U})^\top \\
&= \operatorname{tr}(\widehat{\boldsymbol{\Theta}} - \boldsymbol{\Theta})\boldsymbol{U}\boldsymbol{U}^\top(\widehat{\boldsymbol{\Theta}} - \boldsymbol{\Theta})^\top \neq L_F(\widehat{\boldsymbol{\Theta}}, \theta).
\end{aligned}
$$

We may need to discuss invariance in terms of the original multivariate linear model (4.1), but this is omitted. For invariance in estimation of the covariance matrix, see Chap. 7.

A general theory of invariance and its applications in statistics are discussed by Eaton (1983, 1989). For finding decision-theoretically optimal estimators, it is standard tactics to focus on a restricted class of invariant estimators. See also Lehmann and Casella (1998) for the role of invariance in decision-theoretic estimation.

References

T.W. Anderson, *An Introduction to Multivariate Statistical Analysis*, 3rd edn. (Wiley, New York, 2003)
M.L. Eaton, *Multivariate Statistics: A Vector Space Approach* (Wiley, New York, 1983)
M.L. Eaton, *Group Invariance Application in Statistics*. Regional Conference Series in Probability and Statistics, vol. 1 (Institute of Mathematical Statistics, Hayward, 1989)
E.L. Lehmann, G. Casella, *Theory of Point Estimation*, 2nd edn. (Springer, New York, 1998)
R.J. Muirhead, *Aspects of Multivariate Statistical Theory* (Wiley, New York, 1982)

Chapter 5
A Generalized Stein Identity and Matrix Differential Operators

In shrinkage estimation, the Stein (1973, 1981) identity is known as an integration by parts formula for deriving unbiased risk estimates. It is a simple but very powerful mathematical tool and has contributed significantly to the development of shrinkage estimation. This chapter provides a generalized Stein identity in matrix-variate normal distribution model and also some useful results on matrix differential operators for a unified application of the identity to high- and low-dimensional normal models.

5.1 Stein's Identity in Matrix-Variate Normal Distribution

For $\boldsymbol{X} = (x_{ij}) \in \mathbb{R}^{m\times p}$, denote by $\mathrm{d}_{ij}^X = \partial/\partial x_{ij}$ the differential operator with respect to the (i, j)-th element of $\boldsymbol{X}$. The matrix differential operator with respect to $\boldsymbol{X}$ is defined by $\nabla_X = (\mathrm{d}_{ij}^X)$, which is an $m \times p$ matrix. Let $\boldsymbol{G} = (g_{ij})$ be a $p \times a$ matrix-valued function such that all the elements of $\boldsymbol{G}$, g_{ij}'s, are absolutely continuous functions of $\boldsymbol{X}$. Define $\nabla_X \boldsymbol{G}$ as a usual matrix product: For $i = 1, \ldots, m$ and $j = 1, \ldots, a$, the (i, j)-th element of $\nabla_X \boldsymbol{G}$ is $\{\nabla_X \boldsymbol{G}\}_{ij} = \sum_{k=1}^p \mathrm{d}_{ik}^X g_{kj}$. As for a scalar-valued function f, an $m \times p$ matrix $\nabla_X f(\boldsymbol{X})$ is defined by $\nabla_X f(\boldsymbol{X}) = \nabla_X\{f(\boldsymbol{X})\boldsymbol{I}_p\}$. Then a generalized Stein identity is given in the following theorem.

Theorem 5.1 *Let $\boldsymbol{X} = (x_{ij}) \sim \mathcal{N}_{m\times p}(\boldsymbol{\Theta}, \boldsymbol{\Omega} \otimes \boldsymbol{\Sigma})$, where $\boldsymbol{\Theta} = (\theta_{ij}) \in \mathbb{R}^{m\times p}$, $\boldsymbol{\Omega} \in \mathbb{S}_m^{(+)}$ and $\boldsymbol{\Sigma} \in \mathbb{S}_p^{(+)}$. Let $\boldsymbol{G}_1 \in \mathbb{R}^{a\times m}$ and $\boldsymbol{G}_2 \in \mathbb{R}^{p\times b}$ such that*

(i) all the elements of $\boldsymbol{G}_1$ and $\boldsymbol{G}_2$ are absolutely continuous functions of $\boldsymbol{X}$,
(ii) $E[|\{\boldsymbol{G}_1(\boldsymbol{X} - \boldsymbol{\Theta})\boldsymbol{G}_2\}_{ij}|] < \infty$ for any $i \in \{1, \ldots, a\}$ and $j \in \{1, \ldots, b\}$.

Then

$$E[\boldsymbol{G}_1(\boldsymbol{X} - \boldsymbol{\Theta})\boldsymbol{G}_2] = E[\boldsymbol{G}_1\boldsymbol{\Omega}\nabla_X\boldsymbol{\Sigma}\boldsymbol{G}_2 + (\boldsymbol{G}_2^\top\boldsymbol{\Sigma}\nabla_X^\top\boldsymbol{\Omega}\boldsymbol{G}_1^\top)^\top]. \tag{5.1}$$

H. Tsukuma and T. Kubokawa, *Shrinkage Estimation for Mean and Covariance Matrices*, JSS Research Series in Statistics, https://doi.org/10.1007/978-981-15-1596-5_5

Proof Let $\boldsymbol{\Gamma} = (\gamma_{ij}) \in \mathbb{U}_m$ and $\boldsymbol{\Lambda} = (\lambda_{ij}) \in \mathbb{U}_p$ such that $\boldsymbol{\Omega} = \boldsymbol{\Gamma}\boldsymbol{\Gamma}^\top$ and $\boldsymbol{\Sigma} = \boldsymbol{\Lambda}\boldsymbol{\Lambda}^\top$. Let $\boldsymbol{Z} = (z_{ij}) = \boldsymbol{\Gamma}^{-1}\boldsymbol{X}(\boldsymbol{\Lambda}^\top)^{-1}$ and $\boldsymbol{\Xi} = (\xi_{ij}) = \boldsymbol{\Gamma}^{-1}\boldsymbol{\Theta}(\boldsymbol{\Lambda}^\top)^{-1}$. Note here from Proposition 3.5 that $\boldsymbol{Z} \sim \mathcal{N}_{m\times p}(\boldsymbol{\Xi}, \boldsymbol{I}_m \otimes \boldsymbol{I}_p)$, namely, the z_{ij}'s are independently distributed as $z_{ij} \sim \mathcal{N}(\xi_{ij}, 1)$.

Denote $\boldsymbol{G}_1 = \boldsymbol{G}_1(\boldsymbol{X})$ and $\boldsymbol{G}_2 = \boldsymbol{G}_2(\boldsymbol{X})$. For $i = 1, \dots, a$ and $j = 1, \dots, b$, let h_{ij} be the (i, j)-th element of $E[\boldsymbol{G}_1(\boldsymbol{X} - \boldsymbol{\Theta})\boldsymbol{G}_2]$, which is given by

$$\begin{aligned} h_{ij} &= E[\{\boldsymbol{G}_1(\boldsymbol{\Gamma}\boldsymbol{Z}\boldsymbol{\Lambda}^\top)\boldsymbol{\Gamma}(\boldsymbol{Z} - \boldsymbol{\Xi})\boldsymbol{\Lambda}^\top\boldsymbol{G}_2(\boldsymbol{\Gamma}\boldsymbol{Z}\boldsymbol{\Lambda}^\top)\}_{ij}] \\ &= \sum_{k=1}^{m}\sum_{l=1}^{p} E[\{\boldsymbol{G}_1(\boldsymbol{\Gamma}\boldsymbol{Z}\boldsymbol{\Lambda}^\top)\boldsymbol{\Gamma}\}_{ik}(z_{kl} - \xi_{kl})\{\boldsymbol{\Lambda}^\top\boldsymbol{G}_2(\boldsymbol{\Gamma}\boldsymbol{Z}\boldsymbol{\Lambda}^\top)\}_{lj}]. \end{aligned}$$

By the integration by parts formula, or by the Stein identity (1.3),

$$\begin{aligned} h_{ij} &= \sum_{k=1}^{m}\sum_{l=1}^{p} E\left[\mathrm{d}_{kl}^{Z}\left[\{\boldsymbol{G}_1(\boldsymbol{\Gamma}\boldsymbol{Z}\boldsymbol{\Lambda}^\top)\boldsymbol{\Gamma}\}_{ik}\{\boldsymbol{\Lambda}^\top\boldsymbol{G}_2(\boldsymbol{\Gamma}\boldsymbol{Z}\boldsymbol{\Lambda}^\top)\}_{lj}\right]\right] \\ &= \sum_{k=1}^{m}\sum_{l=1}^{p} E\left[\{\boldsymbol{G}_1(\boldsymbol{\Gamma}\boldsymbol{Z}\boldsymbol{\Lambda}^\top)\boldsymbol{\Gamma}\}_{ik}\mathrm{d}_{kl}^{Z}\{\boldsymbol{\Lambda}^\top\boldsymbol{G}_2(\boldsymbol{\Gamma}\boldsymbol{Z}\boldsymbol{\Lambda}^\top)\}_{lj}\right. \\ &\qquad\qquad \left.+\{\boldsymbol{\Lambda}^\top\boldsymbol{G}_2(\boldsymbol{\Gamma}\boldsymbol{Z}\boldsymbol{\Lambda}^\top)\}_{lj}\mathrm{d}_{kl}^{Z}\{\boldsymbol{G}_1(\boldsymbol{\Gamma}\boldsymbol{Z}\boldsymbol{\Lambda}^\top)\boldsymbol{\Gamma}\}_{ik}\right], \end{aligned}$$

where $\mathrm{d}_{kl}^{Z} = \partial/\partial z_{kl}$. Since $x_{ij} = \{\boldsymbol{\Gamma}\boldsymbol{Z}\boldsymbol{\Lambda}^\top\}_{ij} = \sum_{q=1}^{m}\sum_{r=1}^{p}\gamma_{iq}z_{qr}\lambda_{jr}$, using the chain rule gives

$$\mathrm{d}_{kl}^{Z} = \sum_{i=1}^{m}\sum_{j=1}^{p}\left[\mathrm{d}_{kl}^{Z}x_{ij}\right]\cdot\mathrm{d}_{ij}^{X} = \sum_{i=1}^{m}\sum_{j=1}^{p}\gamma_{ik}\lambda_{jl}\cdot\mathrm{d}_{ij}^{X} = \{\boldsymbol{\Gamma}^\top\nabla_X\boldsymbol{\Lambda}\}_{kl}, \tag{5.2}$$

so that

$$\begin{aligned} h_{ij} &= \sum_{k=1}^{m}\sum_{l=1}^{p} E[\{\boldsymbol{G}_1(\boldsymbol{X})\boldsymbol{\Gamma}\}_{ik}\{\boldsymbol{\Gamma}^\top\nabla_X\boldsymbol{\Lambda}\}_{kl}\{\boldsymbol{\Lambda}^\top\boldsymbol{G}_2(\boldsymbol{X})\}_{lj} \\ &\qquad\qquad + \{\boldsymbol{\Lambda}^\top\boldsymbol{G}_2(\boldsymbol{X})\}_{lj}\{\boldsymbol{\Gamma}^\top\nabla_X\boldsymbol{\Lambda}\}_{kl}\{\boldsymbol{G}_1(\boldsymbol{X})\boldsymbol{\Gamma}\}_{ik}] \\ &= E[\{\boldsymbol{G}_1\boldsymbol{\Gamma}\boldsymbol{\Gamma}^\top\nabla_X\boldsymbol{\Lambda}\boldsymbol{\Lambda}^\top\boldsymbol{G}_2\}_{ij} + \{\boldsymbol{G}_2^\top\boldsymbol{\Lambda}\boldsymbol{\Lambda}^\top\nabla_X^\top\boldsymbol{\Gamma}\boldsymbol{\Gamma}^\top\boldsymbol{G}_1^\top\}_{ji}] \\ &= E[\{\boldsymbol{G}_1\boldsymbol{\Omega}\nabla_X\boldsymbol{\Sigma}\boldsymbol{G}_2\}_{ij} + \{(\boldsymbol{G}_2^\top\boldsymbol{\Sigma}\nabla_X^\top\boldsymbol{\Omega}\boldsymbol{G}_1^\top)^\top\}_{ij}]. \end{aligned}$$

Thus the proof is complete. □

In the proof of Theorem 5.1, the differentiability of elements of $\boldsymbol{G}_1$ and $\boldsymbol{G}_2$ and the interchangeability of integrals are guaranteed, respectively, by conditions (i) and (ii) of Theorem 5.1.

From Theorem 5.1, if $\boldsymbol{X} \sim \mathcal{N}_{m\times p}(\boldsymbol{\Theta}, \boldsymbol{I}_m \otimes \boldsymbol{\Sigma})$ then, under some suitable conditions,

$$E[\operatorname{tr}(\boldsymbol{X}-\boldsymbol{\Theta})\boldsymbol{\Sigma}^{-1}\boldsymbol{G}^\top] = E[\operatorname{tr}\nabla_X \boldsymbol{G}^\top], \tag{5.3}$$

where all the elements of $\boldsymbol{G}$ ($\in \mathbb{R}^{m\times p}$) are absolutely continuous functions of $\boldsymbol{X}$. The r.h.s. of (5.3) depends only on expectations of the diagonals of $\nabla_X \boldsymbol{G}^\top$, but not on those of the off-diagonals. See also Bilodeau and Kariya (1989) and Konno (1992) for Stein-type identities on matrix-variate normal distribution. The appendix of this chapter will discuss a simple derivation of (5.3) via the Gauss divergence theorem.

The Stein identity (5.1), or (5.3), yields a useful identity on the chi-square distribution. Let $\boldsymbol{x} = (x_i) \sim \mathcal{N}_n(\boldsymbol{0}_n, \sigma^2 \boldsymbol{I}_n)$ and let $\nabla_x = (\partial/\partial x_i)$ be the n-dimensional differential operator vector. For a differentiable function $g(s)$ with $s = \|\boldsymbol{x}\|^2$, using the Stein identity leads to

$$E\left[\frac{g(s)}{\sigma^2}\right] = E\left[\boldsymbol{x}^\top \boldsymbol{x}\frac{g(s)}{\sigma^2 s}\right] = E\left[\nabla_x^\top \boldsymbol{x}\frac{g(s)}{s}\right] = E\left[(n-2)\frac{g(s)}{s} + 2g'(s)\right], \tag{5.4}$$

where $g'(s) = \mathrm{d}g(s)/\mathrm{d}s$. Since $s \sim \sigma^2\chi_n^2$, the identity (5.4) is named the chi-square identity, which was derived by Efron and Morris (1976).

The chi-square identity (5.4) can be extended to an identity on the nonsingular Wishart distribution. Let $\boldsymbol{S} = (s_{ij}) \sim \mathcal{W}_p(n, \boldsymbol{\Sigma})$ and let D_S be the $p \times p$ matrix differential operator whose (i, j)-th element is $(1/2)(1+\delta_{ij})(\partial/\partial s_{ij})$, where δ_{ij} represents the Kronecker delta, namely, $\delta_{ij} = 1$ if $i = j$ and $\delta_{ij} = 0$ otherwise. Under suitable conditions, we can obtain an identity

$$E[\operatorname{tr}\boldsymbol{\Sigma}^{-1}\boldsymbol{G}] = E[(n-p-1)\operatorname{tr}\boldsymbol{S}^{-1}\boldsymbol{G} + 2\operatorname{tr}\mathrm{D}_S\boldsymbol{G}], \tag{5.5}$$

where all the elements of $\boldsymbol{G}$ ($\in \mathbb{S}_p$) are absolutely continuous functions of $\boldsymbol{S}$. In the literature, the identity (5.5) is called the Haff (1977, 1979) identity, and it is a useful tool for estimation of $\boldsymbol{\Sigma}$. Clearly, when $p = 1$, the Haff identity (5.5) is equivalent to the chi-square identity (5.4). See the appendix of this chapter for a brief derivation of the Haff identity (5.5).

5.2 Some Useful Results on Matrix Differential Operators

Let $\boldsymbol{Y} = (y_{ab}) \in \mathbb{R}^{n\times p}$. Denote the $n \times p$ matrix differential operator with respect to $\boldsymbol{Y}$ by $\nabla_Y = (\mathrm{d}_{ab}^Y)$ with $\mathrm{d}_{ab}^Y = \partial/\partial y_{ab}$. Here, we provide calculus formulas for $\boldsymbol{S} = (s_{ij}) = \boldsymbol{Y}^\top\boldsymbol{Y} \in \mathbb{S}_{p,\nu}^{(+)}$ with $\nu = n \wedge p$ and its Moore-Penrose inverse $\boldsymbol{S}^+ = (s_{ij}^+)$.

Lemma 5.1 *Abbreviate* d_{ab}^Y *to* d. *Denote* $\mathrm{d}\boldsymbol{S} = (\mathrm{d}s_{ij})$ *and* $\mathrm{d}\boldsymbol{S}^+ = (\mathrm{d}s_{ij}^+)$. *Then*

$$\mathrm{d}\boldsymbol{S}^+ = -\boldsymbol{S}^+[\mathrm{d}\boldsymbol{S}]\boldsymbol{S}^+ + (\boldsymbol{I}_p - \boldsymbol{S}\boldsymbol{S}^+)[\mathrm{d}\boldsymbol{S}]\boldsymbol{S}^+\boldsymbol{S}^+ + \boldsymbol{S}^+\boldsymbol{S}^+[\mathrm{d}\boldsymbol{S}](\boldsymbol{I}_p - \boldsymbol{S}\boldsymbol{S}^+).$$

Proof Note that $\boldsymbol{S}^+ = \boldsymbol{S}^+\boldsymbol{S}\boldsymbol{S}^+$, $\boldsymbol{S}\boldsymbol{S}^+ = \boldsymbol{S}^+\boldsymbol{S}$ and $\boldsymbol{S} = \boldsymbol{S}\boldsymbol{S}\boldsymbol{S}^+$. Differentiating both sides of $\boldsymbol{S}^+ = \boldsymbol{S}^+ \times \boldsymbol{S} \times \boldsymbol{S}^+$, we have $\mathrm{d}\boldsymbol{S}^+ = [\mathrm{d}\boldsymbol{S}^+]\boldsymbol{S}\boldsymbol{S}^+ + \boldsymbol{S}^+[\mathrm{d}\boldsymbol{S}]\boldsymbol{S}^+ + \boldsymbol{S}\boldsymbol{S}^+\mathrm{d}\boldsymbol{S}^+$, so that

$$[\mathrm{d}\boldsymbol{S}^+]\boldsymbol{S}\boldsymbol{S}^+ = -\boldsymbol{S}^+[\mathrm{d}\boldsymbol{S}]\boldsymbol{S}^+ + (\boldsymbol{I}_p - \boldsymbol{S}\boldsymbol{S}^+)\mathrm{d}\boldsymbol{S}^+.$$

Thus

$$\begin{aligned}\mathrm{d}\boldsymbol{S}^+ &= [\mathrm{d}\boldsymbol{S}^+]\{\boldsymbol{S}\boldsymbol{S}^+ + (\boldsymbol{I}_p - \boldsymbol{S}\boldsymbol{S}^+)\}\\ &= [\mathrm{d}\boldsymbol{S}^+]\boldsymbol{S}\boldsymbol{S}^+ + [\mathrm{d}\boldsymbol{S}^+](\boldsymbol{I}_p - \boldsymbol{S}\boldsymbol{S}^+)\\ &= -\boldsymbol{S}^+[\mathrm{d}\boldsymbol{S}]\boldsymbol{S}^+ + (\boldsymbol{I}_p - \boldsymbol{S}\boldsymbol{S}^+)\mathrm{d}\boldsymbol{S}^+ + \{(\boldsymbol{I}_p - \boldsymbol{S}\boldsymbol{S}^+)\mathrm{d}\boldsymbol{S}^+\}^\top. \qquad (5.6)\end{aligned}$$

Differentiating both sides of $\boldsymbol{S} = \boldsymbol{S}\boldsymbol{S}^+ \times \boldsymbol{S}$ yields $\mathrm{d}\boldsymbol{S} = [\mathrm{d}(\boldsymbol{S}\boldsymbol{S}^+)]\boldsymbol{S} + \boldsymbol{S}\boldsymbol{S}^+\mathrm{d}\boldsymbol{S}$, which implies that $[\mathrm{d}(\boldsymbol{S}\boldsymbol{S}^+)]\boldsymbol{S} = (\boldsymbol{I}_p - \boldsymbol{S}\boldsymbol{S}^+)\mathrm{d}\boldsymbol{S}$, which further implies that

$$[\mathrm{d}(\boldsymbol{S}\boldsymbol{S}^+)]\boldsymbol{S}^+ = (\boldsymbol{I}_p - \boldsymbol{S}\boldsymbol{S}^+)[\mathrm{d}\boldsymbol{S}]\boldsymbol{S}^+\boldsymbol{S}^+. \qquad (5.7)$$

Differentiating both sides of $\boldsymbol{S}^+ = \boldsymbol{S}\boldsymbol{S}^+ \times \boldsymbol{S}^+$, we obtain $\mathrm{d}\boldsymbol{S}^+ = [\mathrm{d}(\boldsymbol{S}\boldsymbol{S}^+)]\boldsymbol{S}^+ + \boldsymbol{S}\boldsymbol{S}^+\mathrm{d}\boldsymbol{S}^+$, namely,

$$(\boldsymbol{I}_p - \boldsymbol{S}\boldsymbol{S}^+)\mathrm{d}\boldsymbol{S}^+ = [\mathrm{d}(\boldsymbol{S}\boldsymbol{S}^+)]\boldsymbol{S}^+ = (\boldsymbol{I}_p - \boldsymbol{S}\boldsymbol{S}^+)[\mathrm{d}\boldsymbol{S}]\boldsymbol{S}^+\boldsymbol{S}^+, \qquad (5.8)$$

where the second equality follows from (5.7). Substituting (5.8) into (5.6) completes the proof. □

Lemma 5.2 *Denote the Kronecker delta by δ_{ij}, namely, $\delta_{ij} = 1$ for $i = j$ and $\delta_{ij} = 0$ for $i \neq j$. For $a, i \in \{1, \ldots, n\}$ and $b, j, k \in \{1, \ldots, p\}$, we have*

(i) $\mathrm{d}^Y_{ab} y_{ij} = \delta_{ai}\delta_{bj}$,
(ii) $\mathrm{d}^Y_{ab} s_{jk} = \delta_{bj} y_{ak} + \delta_{bk} y_{aj}$,
(iii) $\mathrm{d}^Y_{ab} s^+_{jk} = -\{\boldsymbol{Y}\boldsymbol{S}^+\}_{ak} s^+_{bj} - \{\boldsymbol{Y}\boldsymbol{S}^+\}_{aj} s^+_{bk} + \{\boldsymbol{Y}\boldsymbol{S}^+\boldsymbol{S}^+\}_{ak}\{\boldsymbol{I}_p - \boldsymbol{S}\boldsymbol{S}^+\}_{bj}$ $+\{\boldsymbol{Y}\boldsymbol{S}^+\boldsymbol{S}^+\}_{aj}\{\boldsymbol{I}_p - \boldsymbol{S}\boldsymbol{S}^+\}_{bk}$,
(iv) $\mathrm{d}^Y_{ab}\{\boldsymbol{Y}\boldsymbol{S}^+\}_{ik} = \{\boldsymbol{I}_n - \boldsymbol{Y}\boldsymbol{S}^+\boldsymbol{Y}^\top\}_{ai} s^+_{bk} + \{\boldsymbol{Y}\boldsymbol{S}^+\boldsymbol{S}^+\boldsymbol{Y}^\top\}_{ai}\{\boldsymbol{I}_p - \boldsymbol{S}\boldsymbol{S}^+\}_{bk}$ $-\{\boldsymbol{Y}\boldsymbol{S}^+\}_{ak}\{\boldsymbol{Y}\boldsymbol{S}^+\}_{ib}$.

Proof Obviously, (i) holds. Differentiating $s_{jk} = \sum_{c=1}^n y_{cj} y_{ck}$ with respect to y_{ab} yields

$$\begin{aligned}\mathrm{d}^Y_{ab} s_{jk} &= \sum_{c=1}^n (y_{ck}\mathrm{d}^Y_{ab} y_{cj} + y_{cj}\mathrm{d}^Y_{ab} y_{ck})\\ &= \sum_{c=1}^n (y_{ck}\delta_{ac}\delta_{bj} + y_{cj}\delta_{ac}\delta_{bk}) = \delta_{bj} y_{ak} + y_{aj}\delta_{bk},\end{aligned}$$

which shows (ii).

From Lemma 5.1 and (ii), it is observed that

$$
\begin{aligned}
\mathrm{d}^Y_{ab} s^+_{jk} &= \{\mathrm{d}^Y_{ab} \boldsymbol{S}^+\}_{jk} \\
&= \sum_{c=1}^{p}\sum_{d=1}^{p}\Big[- s^+_{jc}[\mathrm{d}^Y_{ab} s_{cd}] s^+_{dk} + \{\boldsymbol{I}_p - \boldsymbol{S}\boldsymbol{S}^+\}_{jc}[\mathrm{d}^Y_{ab} s_{cd}]\{\boldsymbol{S}^+\boldsymbol{S}^+\}_{dk} \\
&\qquad + \{\boldsymbol{S}^+\boldsymbol{S}^+\}_{jc}[\mathrm{d}^Y_{ab} s_{cd}]\{\boldsymbol{I}_p - \boldsymbol{S}\boldsymbol{S}^+\}_{dk}\Big] \\
&= -s^+_{bj}\{\boldsymbol{Y}\boldsymbol{S}^+\}_{ak} - \{\boldsymbol{Y}\boldsymbol{S}^+\}_{aj} s^+_{bk} \\
&\quad + \{\boldsymbol{I}_p - \boldsymbol{S}\boldsymbol{S}^+\}_{bj}\{\boldsymbol{Y}\boldsymbol{S}^+\boldsymbol{S}^+\}_{ak} + \{\boldsymbol{Y}(\boldsymbol{I}_p - \boldsymbol{S}\boldsymbol{S}^+)\}_{aj}\{\boldsymbol{S}^+\boldsymbol{S}^+\}_{bk} \\
&\quad + \{\boldsymbol{S}^+\boldsymbol{S}^+\}_{bj}\{\boldsymbol{Y}(\boldsymbol{I}_p - \boldsymbol{S}\boldsymbol{S}^+)\}_{ak} + \{\boldsymbol{Y}\boldsymbol{S}^+\boldsymbol{S}^+\}_{aj}\{\boldsymbol{I}_p - \boldsymbol{S}\boldsymbol{S}^+\}_{bk}.
\end{aligned}
$$

Noting that $\boldsymbol{Y}(\boldsymbol{I}_p - \boldsymbol{S}\boldsymbol{S}^+) = \boldsymbol{0}_{n\times p}$ gives (iii).

In view of the product rule,

$$
\mathrm{d}^Y_{ab}\{\boldsymbol{Y}\boldsymbol{S}^+\}_{ik} = \sum_{c=1}^{p}\big[[\mathrm{d}^Y_{ab} y_{ic}] s^+_{ck} + y_{ic}\mathrm{d}^Y_{ab} s^+_{ck}\big].
$$

Using (i) and (iii) and subsequently summing over all c, we obtain (iv). □

The following lemma is useful in estimation of a covariance matrix in multivariate normal distribution model. The proof of the lemma is similar to that of the $p > n$ case given in Konno (2009). See also Stein (1977), Sheena (1995) and Kubokawa and Srivastava (2008).

Lemma 5.3 *Denote by* $\boldsymbol{S} = \boldsymbol{H}\boldsymbol{L}\boldsymbol{H}^\top$ *the eigenvalue decomposition of* $\boldsymbol{S} = \boldsymbol{Y}^\top\boldsymbol{Y}$, *where* $\boldsymbol{L} = \mathrm{diag}\,(\ell_1, \ldots, \ell_\nu) \in \mathbb{D}^{(\geq 0)}_\nu$ *and* $\boldsymbol{H} \in \mathbb{V}_{p,\nu}$ *with* $\nu = n \wedge p$. *Let* $\boldsymbol{\Phi} = \mathrm{diag}\,(\phi_1, \ldots, \phi_\nu) \in \mathbb{D}_\nu$ *such that all the diagonal elements* ϕ_i*'s are differentiable functions of* $\boldsymbol{L}$. *Then*

$$
\nabla^\top_Y \boldsymbol{Y}\boldsymbol{S}^+\boldsymbol{H}\boldsymbol{\Phi}\boldsymbol{H}^\top = \boldsymbol{H}\boldsymbol{\Phi}^*\boldsymbol{H}^\top + (\mathrm{tr}\,\boldsymbol{L}^{-1}\boldsymbol{\Phi})(\boldsymbol{I}_p - \boldsymbol{H}\boldsymbol{H}^\top),
$$

where $\boldsymbol{\Phi}^* = \mathrm{diag}\,(\phi^*_1, \ldots, \phi^*_\nu)$ *and for* $i = 1, \ldots, \nu$

$$
\phi^*_i = (n - \nu - 1)\frac{\phi_i}{\ell_i} + 2\frac{\partial \phi_i}{\partial \ell_i} + \sum_{j\neq i}^{\nu}\frac{\phi_i - \phi_j}{\ell_i - \ell_j}.
$$

In particular,

$$
\mathrm{tr}\,\nabla^\top_Y \boldsymbol{Y}\boldsymbol{S}^+\boldsymbol{H}\boldsymbol{\Phi}\boldsymbol{H}^\top = \sum_{i=1}^{\nu}\left\{(|n - p| - 1)\frac{\phi_i}{\ell_i} + 2\frac{\partial \phi_i}{\partial \ell_i} + 2\sum_{j>i}^{\nu}\frac{\phi_i - \phi_j}{\ell_i - \ell_j}\right\}.
$$

Appendix

In this appendix, we first give another derivation of the Stein identity (5.3). Denote by $f(\boldsymbol{X})$ the p.d.f. of $\mathcal{N}_{m\times p}(\boldsymbol{\Theta}, \boldsymbol{I}_m \otimes \boldsymbol{\Sigma})$. Let

$$I_{ST}(\boldsymbol{G}) = \int_{\mathbb{R}^{m\times p}} \mathrm{tr}\, \nabla_X\{\boldsymbol{G}^\top f(\boldsymbol{X})\}(\mathrm{d}\boldsymbol{X}).$$

It follows that $\nabla_X f(\boldsymbol{X}) = -(\boldsymbol{X} - \boldsymbol{\Theta})\boldsymbol{\Sigma}^{-1} f(\boldsymbol{X})$, so that

$$I_{ST}(\boldsymbol{G}) = E[\,\mathrm{tr}\, \nabla_X \boldsymbol{G}^\top] - E[\,\mathrm{tr}\,(\boldsymbol{X} - \boldsymbol{\Theta})\boldsymbol{\Sigma}^{-1}\boldsymbol{G}^\top]$$

provided the expectations exist. Hence the Stein identity (5.3) can be verified if $I_{ST}(\boldsymbol{G}) = 0$.

For $r > 0$, let $\mathbb{B}_r = \{\boldsymbol{X} \in \mathbb{R}^{m\times p} : \|\mathrm{vec}(\boldsymbol{X})\| \le r\}$, where $\|\cdot\|$ is the usual Euclidean norm and $\mathrm{vec}(\cdot)$ is defined in Definition 2.3. Then $\mathbb{B}_r \to \mathbb{R}^{m\times p}$ as $r \to \infty$ and

$$I_{ST}(\boldsymbol{G}) = \lim_{r\to\infty} \int_{\mathbb{B}_r} \mathrm{vec}(\nabla_X)^\top \mathrm{vec}(\boldsymbol{G} f(\boldsymbol{X}))(\mathrm{d}\boldsymbol{X}).$$

The boundary of $\mathbb{B}_r$ is expressed by $\partial\mathbb{B}_r = \{\mathrm{vec}(\boldsymbol{X}) \in \mathbb{R}^{mp} : \|\mathrm{vec}(\boldsymbol{X})\| = r\}$. Denote by $\boldsymbol{u}$ an outward unit normal vector at a point $\mathrm{vec}(\boldsymbol{X}) \in \partial\mathbb{B}_r$. Let $\lambda_{\partial\mathbb{B}_r}$ be Lebesgue measure on $\partial\mathbb{B}_r$. By the Gauss divergence theorem,

$$I_{ST}(\boldsymbol{G}) = \lim_{r\to\infty} \int_{\partial\mathbb{B}_r} \boldsymbol{u}^\top \mathrm{vec}(\boldsymbol{G}) f(\boldsymbol{X})(\mathrm{d}\lambda_{\partial\mathbb{B}_r}).$$

For details of the Gauss divergence theorem, see Fleming (1977).

Let $o(\cdot)$ be the Landau symbol, namely, for real-valued functions $f(x)$ and $g(x)$ with $g(x) \neq 0$, we write $f(x) = o(g(x))$ when $\lim_{x\to c} |f(x)/g(x)| = 0$ for an extended real number c. If

$$\sup_{\mathrm{vec}(\boldsymbol{X})\in\partial\mathbb{B}_r} \|\mathrm{vec}(\boldsymbol{G})\| f(\boldsymbol{X}) = o(r^{1-mp}) \quad \text{as } r \to \infty,$$

then $I_{ST}(\boldsymbol{G}) = 0$. In fact,

$$\begin{aligned}\int_{\partial\mathbb{B}_r} |\boldsymbol{u}^\top \mathrm{vec}(\boldsymbol{G})| f(\boldsymbol{X})(\mathrm{d}\lambda_{\partial\mathbb{B}_r}) &\le \int_{\partial\mathbb{B}_r} \|\mathrm{vec}(\boldsymbol{G})\| f(\boldsymbol{X})(\mathrm{d}\lambda_{\partial\mathbb{B}_r}) \\ &\le o(r^{1-mp}) \int_{\partial\mathbb{B}_r} (\mathrm{d}\lambda_{\partial\mathbb{B}_r}) = o(1),\end{aligned}$$

because $\int_{\partial\mathbb{B}_r} (\mathrm{d}\lambda_{\partial\mathbb{B}_r})$ is the surface area of the $(mp-1)$-sphere of radius r in $\mathbb{R}^{mp}$, namely, $\int_{\partial\mathbb{B}_r} (\mathrm{d}\lambda_{\partial\mathbb{B}_r}) \approx r^{mp-1}$.

Next, a simple derivation of the Haff identity (5.5) is provided by using the Gauss divergence theorem. The derivation is essentially the same as Haff (1977, 1979). Let $f(\boldsymbol{S})$ be the p.d.f. of $\mathcal{W}_p(n, \boldsymbol{\Sigma})$. For a differentiable matrix-valued function $\boldsymbol{G} \in \mathbb{S}_p$, let

$$I_{HF}(\boldsymbol{G}) = \int_{\mathbb{S}_p^{(+)}} \operatorname{tr} \mathrm{D}_S\{\boldsymbol{G} f(\boldsymbol{S})\}(\mathrm{d}\boldsymbol{S})$$

Since $\mathrm{D}_S|\boldsymbol{S}| = \boldsymbol{S}^{-1}|\boldsymbol{S}|$ and $\mathrm{D}_S \operatorname{tr} \boldsymbol{\Sigma}^{-1}\boldsymbol{S} = \boldsymbol{\Sigma}^{-1}$, we get $\mathrm{D}_S f(\boldsymbol{S}) = \{(n-p-1)\boldsymbol{S}^{-1} - \boldsymbol{\Sigma}^{-1}\}f(\boldsymbol{S})/2$, implying that

$$I_{HF}(\boldsymbol{G}) = E[\operatorname{tr} \mathrm{D}_S\boldsymbol{G}] + \frac{n-p-1}{2}E[\operatorname{tr} \boldsymbol{S}^{-1}\boldsymbol{G}] - \frac{1}{2}E[\operatorname{tr} \boldsymbol{\Sigma}^{-1}\boldsymbol{G}]$$

provided the expectations exist. Hence the Haff identity (5.5) follows if $I_{HF}(\boldsymbol{G}) = 0$.

Denote by $\partial/\partial\boldsymbol{S} = (\partial/\partial s_{ij})$ the $p \times p$ matrix differential operator with respect to $\boldsymbol{S} \in \mathbb{S}_p$. For $\boldsymbol{A} = (a_{ij}) \in \mathbb{S}_p$, define

$$\mathrm{Vec}(\boldsymbol{A}) = (a_{11}, a_{21}, \ldots, a_{p1}, a_{22}, a_{32}, \ldots, a_{p2}, \ldots, a_{p-1,p-1}, a_{p,p-1}, a_{pp})^\top \in \mathbb{R}^q,$$

where $q = p(p+1)/2$. From symmetry of $\boldsymbol{G}$, it holds that

$$\begin{aligned}\operatorname{tr} \mathrm{D}_S\{\boldsymbol{G} f(\boldsymbol{S})\} &= \sum_{i=1}^{p}\sum_{j=1}^{p}\frac{1+\delta_{ij}}{2}\frac{\partial}{\partial s_{ij}}\{g_{ji} f(\boldsymbol{S})\} = \sum_{i=1}^{p}\sum_{j=1}^{i}\frac{\partial}{\partial s_{ij}}\{g_{ij} f(\boldsymbol{S})\}\\ &= \mathrm{Vec}(\partial/\partial\boldsymbol{S})^\top \mathrm{Vec}(\boldsymbol{G} f(\boldsymbol{S})),\end{aligned}$$

so that

$$I_{HF}(\boldsymbol{G}) = \int_{\mathbb{S}_p^{(+)}} \mathrm{Vec}(\partial/\partial\boldsymbol{S})^\top \mathrm{Vec}(\boldsymbol{G} f(\boldsymbol{S}))(\mathrm{d}\boldsymbol{S}).$$

For $r > 0$, let $\partial\mathbb{B}_r^q = \{\mathrm{Vec}(\boldsymbol{S}) \in \mathbb{R}^q : \|\mathrm{Vec}(\boldsymbol{S})\| = r\}$ and, for $0 < r_1 \le r_2 < \infty$, let $\mathbb{C}_{r_1,r_2} = \{\mathrm{Vec}(\boldsymbol{S}) \in \mathbb{R}^q : r_1 \le \|\mathrm{Vec}(\boldsymbol{S})\| \le r_2\}$. Then $\mathbb{C}_{r_1,r_2} \cap \mathbb{S}_p^{(+)} \to \mathbb{S}_p^{(+)}$ as $r_1 \to 0$ and $r_2 \to \infty$. The boundary of $\mathbb{C}_{r_1,r_2} \cap \mathbb{S}_p^{(+)}$ can be expressed as $\bigcup_{i=1}^3 \partial\mathbb{B}_i$, where $\partial\mathbb{B}_1$, $\partial\mathbb{B}_2$ and $\partial\mathbb{B}_3$ are certain sets satisfying $\partial\mathbb{B}_1 \subset \partial\mathbb{B}_{r_1}^q$, $\partial\mathbb{B}_2 \subset \partial\mathbb{B}_{r_2}^q$ and $\partial\mathbb{B}_3 \subset \partial\mathbb{S}_p^{(+)}$. Note that, for any point $\boldsymbol{S} \in \partial\mathbb{S}_p^{(+)}$, $|\boldsymbol{S}| = 0$, namely, $f(\boldsymbol{S}) = 0$ when $n - p - 1 > 0$. Let $\boldsymbol{u}_1 = -\mathrm{Vec}(\boldsymbol{S})/\|\mathrm{Vec}(\boldsymbol{S})\|$ for $\mathrm{Vec}(\boldsymbol{S}) \in \partial\mathbb{B}_{r_1}^q$ and $\boldsymbol{u}_2 = \mathrm{Vec}(\boldsymbol{S})/\|\mathrm{Vec}(\boldsymbol{S})\|$ for $\mathrm{Vec}(\boldsymbol{S}) \in \partial\mathbb{B}_{r_2}^q$. Denote by $\lambda_{\partial\mathbb{B}_r^q}$ Lebesgue measure on $\partial\mathbb{B}_r^q$. Using the Gauss divergence theorem gives

$$I_{HF}(\boldsymbol{G}) = \lim_{r_1\to 0}\int_{\partial\mathbb{B}_1} \boldsymbol{u}_1^\top \mathrm{Vec}(\boldsymbol{G}) f(\boldsymbol{S})(\mathrm{d}\lambda_{\partial\mathbb{B}_{r_1}^q}) + \lim_{r_2\to\infty}\int_{\partial\mathbb{B}_2} \boldsymbol{u}_2^\top \mathrm{Vec}(\boldsymbol{G}) f(\boldsymbol{S})(\mathrm{d}\lambda_{\partial\mathbb{B}_{r_2}^q}).$$

Using the Landau symbol $o(\cdot)$, we assume that

$$\sup_{\mathrm{Vec}(\boldsymbol{S})\in\partial\mathbb{B}_1} \|\mathrm{Vec}(\boldsymbol{G})\| f(\boldsymbol{S}) = o(r_1^{1-q}) \quad \text{as } r_1 \to 0$$

and

$$\sup_{\mathrm{Vec}(\boldsymbol{S})\in\partial\mathbb{B}_2} \|\mathrm{Vec}(\boldsymbol{G})\| f(\boldsymbol{S}) = o(r_2^{1-q}) \quad \text{as } r_2 \to \infty.$$

Under these assumptions, we can see that

$$\begin{aligned}\int_{\partial\mathbb{B}_1} |\boldsymbol{u}_1^\top \mathrm{Vec}(\boldsymbol{G})| f(\boldsymbol{S})(\mathrm{d}\lambda_{\partial\mathbb{B}^q_{r_1}}) &\le \int_{\partial\mathbb{B}_1} \|\mathrm{Vec}(\boldsymbol{G})\| f(\boldsymbol{S})(\mathrm{d}\lambda_{\partial\mathbb{B}^q_{r_1}}) \\ &\le o(r_1^{1-q}) \int_{\partial\mathbb{B}^q_{r_1}} (\mathrm{d}\lambda_{\partial\mathbb{B}^q_{r_1}}) = o(1) \qquad \text{as } r_1 \to 0\end{aligned}$$

and also

$$\int_{\partial\mathbb{B}_2} |\boldsymbol{u}_2^\top \mathrm{Vec}(\boldsymbol{G})| f(\boldsymbol{S})(\mathrm{d}\lambda_{\partial\mathbb{B}^q_{r_2}}) \le o(r_2^{1-q}) \int_{\partial\mathbb{B}^q_{r_2}} (\mathrm{d}\lambda_{\partial\mathbb{B}^q_{r_2}}) = o(1) \qquad \text{as } r_2 \to \infty,$$

so that $I_{HF}(\boldsymbol{G}) = 0$.

References

M. Bilodeau, T. Kariya, Minimax estimators in the normal MANOVA model. J. Multivar. Anal. **28**, 260–270 (1989)

B. Efron, C. Morris, Families of minimax estimators of the mean of a multivariate normal distribution. Ann. Stat. **4**, 11–21 (1976)

W. Fleming, *Functions of Several Variables*, 2nd edn. (Springer, New York, 1977)

L.R. Haff, Minimax estimators for a multinormal precision matrix. J. Multivar. Anal. **7**, 374–385 (1977)

L.R. Haff, An identity for the Wishart distribution with applications. J. Multivar. Anal. **9**, 531–544 (1979)

Y. Konno, Improved estimation of matrix of normal mean and eigenvalues in the multivariate F-distribution. Doctoral dissertation, Institute of Mathematics, University of Tsukuba, 1992. http://mcm-www.jwu.ac.jp/~konno/

Y. Konno, Shrinkage estimators for large covariance matrices in multivariate real and complex normal distributions under an invariant quadratic loss. J. Multivar. Anal. **100**, 2237–2253 (2009)

T. Kubokawa, M.S. Srivastava, Estimation of the precision matrix of a singular Wishart distribution and its application in high-dimensional data. J. Multivar. Anal. **99**, 1906–1928 (2008)

Y. Sheena, Unbiased estimator of risk for an orthogonally invariant estimator of a covariance matrix. J. Jpn. Stat. Soc. **25**, 35–48 (1995)

C. Stein, Estimation of the mean of a multivariate normal distribution. Technical Reports No.48 (Department of Statistics, Stanford University, Stanford, 1973)

C. Stein, Lectures on the theory of estimation of many parameters, in *Proceedings of Scientific Seminars of the Steklov Institute Studies in the Statistical Theory of Estimation, Part I*, vol. 74, ed. by I.A. Ibragimov, M.S. Nikulin (Leningrad Division, 1977), pp. 4–65

C. Stein, Estimation of the mean of a multivariate normal distribution. Ann. Stat. **9**, 1135–1151 (1981)

Chapter 6
Estimation of the Mean Matrix

This chapter introduces a unified approach to high- and low-dimensional cases for matricial shrinkage estimation of a normal mean matrix with unknown covariance matrix. A historical background is briefly explained and matricial shrinkage estimators are motivated from an empirical Bayes method. An unbiased risk estimate is unifiedly developed for a class of estimators corresponding to all possible orderings of sample size and dimensions. Specific examples of matricial shrinkage estimators are provided and also some related topics are discussed.

6.1 Introduction

Matricial shrinkage estimation of a mean matrix of a matrix-variate normal distribution has been studied since Efron and Morris (1972, 1976) and Stein (1973). Assume now that an $m \times p$ observed data matrix $\boldsymbol{X}$ follows $\mathcal{N}_{m\times p}(\Xi, \boldsymbol{I}_m \otimes \boldsymbol{I}_p)$, where $p \geq m$ and Ξ is unknown, and consider estimation of the mean matrix Ξ. The performance of its estimator $\widehat{\Xi}$ is evaluated by a risk function relative to the squared Frobenius norm loss

$$L_F(\widehat{\Xi}, \Xi) = \|\widehat{\Xi} - \Xi\|_F^2 = \operatorname{tr}(\widehat{\Xi} - \Xi)(\widehat{\Xi} - \Xi)^\top.$$

The maximum likelihood (ML) estimator of Ξ is $\widehat{\Xi}^{ML} = \boldsymbol{X}$. It is unbiased and minimax. Efron and Morris (1972) considered empirical Bayes estimation for Ξ and showed that $\widehat{\Xi}^{ML}$ is dominated by the resulting empirical Bayes estimator of the form

$$\widehat{\Xi}^{EM} = \{\boldsymbol{I}_m - c_0(\boldsymbol{X}\boldsymbol{X}^\top)^{-1}\}\boldsymbol{X}, \quad c_0 = p - m - 1. \tag{6.1}$$

H. Tsukuma and T. Kubokawa, *Shrinkage Estimation for Mean and Covariance Matrices*, JSS Research Series in Statistics, https://doi.org/10.1007/978-981-15-1596-5_6

This is equivalent to $\{\boldsymbol{I}_m - c_0(\boldsymbol{X}\boldsymbol{X}^\top)^{-1}\}\widehat{\boldsymbol{\Xi}}^{ML}$, which is a matrix multiple of $\widehat{\boldsymbol{\Xi}}^{ML}$, while the James-Stein (1961) type shrinkage estimator can be defined by

$$\widehat{\boldsymbol{\Xi}}^{JS} = \left(1 - \frac{mp-2}{\|\boldsymbol{X}\|_F^2}\right)\widehat{\boldsymbol{\Xi}}^{ML} = \left(1 - \frac{mp-2}{\operatorname{tr}\boldsymbol{X}\boldsymbol{X}^\top}\right)\widehat{\boldsymbol{\Xi}}^{ML},$$

which is a scalar multiple of $\widehat{\boldsymbol{\Xi}}^{ML}$. Therefore $\widehat{\boldsymbol{\Xi}}^{EM}$ and $\widehat{\boldsymbol{\Xi}}^{JS}$ are called, respectively, matricial and scalar shrinkage estimators.

The Efron-Morris estimator $\widehat{\boldsymbol{\Xi}}^{EM}$ can be written as $\widehat{\boldsymbol{\Xi}}^{EM} = (\boldsymbol{I}_m - c_0\boldsymbol{B}\boldsymbol{L}^{-1}\boldsymbol{B}^\top)\boldsymbol{X}$, where $\boldsymbol{X}\boldsymbol{X}^\top = \boldsymbol{B}\boldsymbol{L}\boldsymbol{B}^\top$ such that $\boldsymbol{L} = \operatorname{diag}(l_1, \dots, l_m) \in \mathbb{D}_m^{(\geq 0)}$ and $\boldsymbol{B} \in \mathbb{O}_m$. Efron and Morris (1972) also pointed out an interesting relationship between the mean matrix estimation and estimating a restricted precision matrix. The relationship suggests a positive-part rule for $\widehat{\boldsymbol{\Xi}}^{EM}$ and in fact they showed that

$$\widehat{\boldsymbol{\Xi}}^{PEM} = (\boldsymbol{I}_m - \boldsymbol{B}\boldsymbol{C}\boldsymbol{L}^{-1}\boldsymbol{B}^\top)\boldsymbol{X}, \quad \boldsymbol{C} = \operatorname{diag}(c_1, \dots, c_m), \quad c_i = \min(l_i, c_0), \tag{6.2}$$

dominates $\widehat{\boldsymbol{\Xi}}^{EM}$ under the L_F-loss. Efron and Morris (1976) presented another improved estimator of the form

$$\widehat{\boldsymbol{\Xi}}^{MEM} = \widehat{\boldsymbol{\Xi}}^{EM} - \frac{(m-1)(m+2)}{\|\boldsymbol{X}\|_F^2}\boldsymbol{X}, \tag{6.3}$$

which is uniformly better than $\widehat{\boldsymbol{\Xi}}^{EM}$ under the L_F-loss. Meanwhile, Stein (1973) considered a multivariate generalization of Baranchik's (1970) estimator for a mean vector of multivariate normal distribution. Stein's class of estimators is given by

$$\widehat{\boldsymbol{\Xi}}_\Phi = \{\boldsymbol{I}_m - \boldsymbol{B}\boldsymbol{\Phi}(\boldsymbol{L})\boldsymbol{B}^\top\}\boldsymbol{X}, \quad \boldsymbol{\Phi}(\boldsymbol{L}) = \operatorname{diag}(\phi_1(\boldsymbol{L}), \dots, \phi_m(\boldsymbol{L})), \tag{6.4}$$

where the diagonals of $\boldsymbol{\Phi}(\boldsymbol{L})$ are functions of $\boldsymbol{L}$. Stein (1973) derived an unbiased risk estimate of $\widehat{\boldsymbol{\Xi}}_\Phi$ to provide alternative estimators. For example, he proposed

$$\widehat{\boldsymbol{\Xi}}^{ST} = (\boldsymbol{I}_m - \boldsymbol{B}\boldsymbol{D}\boldsymbol{L}^{-1}\boldsymbol{B}^\top)\boldsymbol{X}, \quad \boldsymbol{D} = \operatorname{diag}(d_1, \dots, d_m), \quad d_i = m + p - 2i - 1, \tag{6.5}$$

which dominates $\widehat{\boldsymbol{\Xi}}^{EM}$ relative to the L_F-loss.

The purpose of this chapter is to extend these results above to the unknown covariance case: Assume that $\boldsymbol{X}$ and $\boldsymbol{Y}$ are mutually independent random matrices distributed as, respectively,

$$\boldsymbol{X} \sim \mathcal{N}_{m\times p}(\boldsymbol{\Theta}, \boldsymbol{I}_m \otimes \boldsymbol{\Sigma}), \qquad \boldsymbol{Y} \sim \mathcal{N}_{n\times p}(\boldsymbol{0}_{n\times p}, \boldsymbol{I}_n \otimes \boldsymbol{\Sigma}), \tag{6.6}$$

where $\boldsymbol{\Theta} \in \mathbb{R}^{m\times p}$ and $\boldsymbol{\Sigma} \in \mathbb{S}_p^{(+)}$ are unknown. The model (6.6) is a canonical form of the multivariate linear regression model (4.1). Denote by $\widehat{\boldsymbol{\Theta}}$ an estimator based on

$\boldsymbol{X}$ and $\boldsymbol{S} = \boldsymbol{Y}^\top \boldsymbol{Y}$. The problem we consider in this chapter is estimation of the mean matrix $\boldsymbol{\Theta}$ relative to invariant quadratic loss

$$L(\widehat{\boldsymbol{\Theta}}, \boldsymbol{\Theta}|\boldsymbol{\Sigma}) = \operatorname{tr}(\widehat{\boldsymbol{\Theta}} - \boldsymbol{\Theta})\boldsymbol{\Sigma}^{-1}(\widehat{\boldsymbol{\Theta}} - \boldsymbol{\Theta})^\top. \tag{6.7}$$

The invariance of (6.7) follows under (4.4) and, more generally, under the group of transformations $\widehat{\boldsymbol{\Theta}} \to \boldsymbol{O}\widehat{\boldsymbol{\Theta}}\boldsymbol{U} + \boldsymbol{A}$, $\boldsymbol{\Theta} \to \boldsymbol{O}\boldsymbol{\Theta}\boldsymbol{U} + \boldsymbol{A}$ and $\boldsymbol{\Sigma} \to \boldsymbol{U}^\top\boldsymbol{\Sigma}\boldsymbol{U}$ for any $\boldsymbol{O} \in \mathbb{O}_m$, $\boldsymbol{U} \in \mathbb{U}_p$ and $\boldsymbol{A} \in \mathbb{R}^{m\times p}$. The performance of $\widehat{\boldsymbol{\Theta}}$ is measured by the risk function $R(\widehat{\boldsymbol{\Theta}}, \boldsymbol{\Theta}) = E[L(\widehat{\boldsymbol{\Theta}}, \boldsymbol{\Theta}|\boldsymbol{\Sigma})]$, where E is expectation taken with respect to (6.6).

The ML estimator of $\boldsymbol{\Theta}$ in (6.6) is $\widehat{\boldsymbol{\Theta}}^{ML} = \boldsymbol{X}$, which is a minimax estimator with the constant risk mp. Thus all estimators dominating $\widehat{\boldsymbol{\Theta}}^{ML}$ are minimax relative to the quadratic loss (6.7). When $n \geq p$ in (6.6) and then the Wishart matrix $\boldsymbol{S}$ is nonsingular with probability one, some studies of improving $\widehat{\boldsymbol{\Theta}}^{ML}$ via matricial shrinkage estimation can be found in Bilodeau and Kariya (1989), Honda (1991), Konno (1990, 1991, 1992) and Tsukuma and Kubokawa (2007). Bilodeau and Kariya (1989) and Konno (1992) studied general classes of matricial shrinkage estimators which can be regarded as an extension of (6.4). In particular, Konno's (1992) class has the form

$$\widehat{\boldsymbol{\Theta}}^K = \begin{cases} \boldsymbol{X}\{\boldsymbol{I}_p - \boldsymbol{Q}\boldsymbol{\Psi}(\boldsymbol{F})\boldsymbol{Q}^{-1}\} & \text{for } m > p, \\ \{\boldsymbol{I}_m - \boldsymbol{R}\boldsymbol{\Psi}(\boldsymbol{F})\boldsymbol{R}^\top\}\boldsymbol{X} & \text{for } p \geq m, \end{cases} \tag{6.8}$$

where $\boldsymbol{F} \in \mathbb{D}^{(\geq 0)}_{m\wedge p}$, $\boldsymbol{Q} \in \mathbb{U}_p$ and $\boldsymbol{R} \in \mathbb{O}_m$ satisfy

$$\begin{cases} \boldsymbol{Q}^\top\boldsymbol{S}\boldsymbol{Q} = \boldsymbol{I}_p \text{ and } \boldsymbol{Q}^\top\boldsymbol{X}^\top\boldsymbol{X}\boldsymbol{Q} = \boldsymbol{F} & \text{for } m > p, \\ \boldsymbol{X}\boldsymbol{S}^{-1}\boldsymbol{X}^\top = \boldsymbol{R}\boldsymbol{F}\boldsymbol{R}^\top & \text{for } p \geq m, \end{cases}$$

and $\boldsymbol{\Psi}(\boldsymbol{F}) \in \mathbb{D}_{m\wedge p}$ whose diagonal elements are functions of $\boldsymbol{F}$. Konno (1992) showed that an unbiased risk estimate of the class (6.8) is only a function of $\boldsymbol{F}$ for both cases of $m > p$ and $p \geq m$. Numerical comparison of shrinkage estimators has been carried out by Tsukuma and Kubokawa (2007). The numerical results suggest that when true eigenvalues of $\boldsymbol{\Sigma}^{-1}\boldsymbol{\Theta}^\top\boldsymbol{\Theta}$ are scattered, matricial shrinkage estimators outperform a James-Stein (1961) type scalar one, which may motivate us to study matricial shrinkage estimation.

This chapter is based in part on Tsukuma and Kubokawa (2015). The structure of this chapter is as follows. In Sect. 6.2, via an empirical Bayes method, we begin by deriving a unified Efron-Morris estimator for any possible ordering on m, p and n. Section 6.3 yields a unified class of matricial shrinkage estimators from the class (6.8) and studies some properties of the unified class. In Sect. 6.4 we derive an unbiased risk estimate of the unified class, and Sect. 6.5 gives specific examples of matricial shrinkage estimators. Section 6.6 discusses some related topics including a method of positive-part rule and an extension to the GMANOVA model. In the Appendix, we supplement some results on matrix differential operators.

6.2 The Unified Efron-Morris Type Estimators Including Singular Cases

6.2.1 Empirical Bayes Methods

First, when $n \geq p$, namely, when $\boldsymbol{S} = \boldsymbol{Y}^\top \boldsymbol{Y}$ is nonsingular, we will derive empirical Bayes estimators of $\boldsymbol{\Theta}$ in (6.6) individually in the cases of $m > p$ and $p \geq m$.

In the case of $m > p$, the prior distribution of $\boldsymbol{\Theta}$ is assumed to be $\mathcal{N}_{m\times p}(\boldsymbol{0}_{m\times p}, \boldsymbol{I}_m \otimes \boldsymbol{A})$, where $\boldsymbol{A} \in \mathbb{S}_p^{(+)}$ is unknown. Then the posterior distribution of $\boldsymbol{\Theta}$ and the marginal distribution of $\boldsymbol{X}$ are, respectively,

$$\boldsymbol{\Theta}|\boldsymbol{X} \sim \mathcal{N}_{m\times p}(\boldsymbol{X}(\boldsymbol{I}_p - \boldsymbol{\Omega}), \boldsymbol{I}_m \otimes (\boldsymbol{\Sigma}^{-1} + \boldsymbol{A}^{-1})^{-1}),$$
$$\boldsymbol{X} \sim \mathcal{N}_{m\times p}(\boldsymbol{0}_{m\times p}, \boldsymbol{I}_m \otimes (\boldsymbol{\Sigma} + \boldsymbol{A})),$$

where $\boldsymbol{\Omega} = (\boldsymbol{\Sigma} + \boldsymbol{A})^{-1}\boldsymbol{\Sigma}$. Thus the posterior mean of $\boldsymbol{\Theta}$ is $\widehat{\boldsymbol{\Theta}}^B = \boldsymbol{X}(\boldsymbol{I}_p - \boldsymbol{\Omega})$. Since $\boldsymbol{\Omega}$ is unknown, it may be estimated from the marginal distributions of $\boldsymbol{S}$ and $\boldsymbol{W} = \boldsymbol{X}^\top \boldsymbol{X}$, which are given by $\boldsymbol{S} \sim \mathcal{W}_p(n, \boldsymbol{\Sigma})$ and $\boldsymbol{W} \sim \mathcal{W}_p(m, \boldsymbol{\Sigma} + \boldsymbol{A})$, respectively. It is reasonable that, as an estimator of $\boldsymbol{\Omega}$, we take $\widehat{\boldsymbol{\Omega}} = c\boldsymbol{W}^{-1}\boldsymbol{S}$ for a suitable constant c. Substituting $\widehat{\boldsymbol{\Omega}}$ for $\boldsymbol{\Omega}$ in $\widehat{\boldsymbol{\Theta}}^B$ yields an Efron-Morris (1972) type empirical Bayes estimator of the form

$$\widehat{\boldsymbol{\Theta}}_1^{EMK} = \boldsymbol{X}(\boldsymbol{I}_p - \widehat{\boldsymbol{\Omega}}) = \boldsymbol{X}\{\boldsymbol{I}_p - c(\boldsymbol{X}^\top \boldsymbol{X})^{-1}\boldsymbol{S}\}.$$

Next, we treat the case of $p \geq m$. Assume that the prior distribution of $\boldsymbol{\Theta}$ is $\mathcal{N}_{m\times p}(\boldsymbol{0}_{m\times p}, \boldsymbol{B} \otimes \boldsymbol{\Sigma})$, where $\boldsymbol{B} \in \mathbb{S}_m^{(+)}$ is unknown. Then the posterior distribution of $\boldsymbol{\Theta}$ and the marginal distribution of $\boldsymbol{X}$ are, respectively,

$$\boldsymbol{\Theta}|\boldsymbol{X} \sim \mathcal{N}_{m\times p}((\boldsymbol{I}_m - \boldsymbol{\Omega})\boldsymbol{X}, (\boldsymbol{I}_m - \boldsymbol{\Omega}) \otimes \boldsymbol{\Sigma}),$$
$$\boldsymbol{X} \sim \mathcal{N}_{m\times p}(\boldsymbol{0}_{m\times p}, \boldsymbol{\Omega}^{-1} \otimes \boldsymbol{\Sigma}),$$

where $\boldsymbol{\Omega} = (\boldsymbol{I}_m + \boldsymbol{B})^{-1}$. The resulting posterior mean of $\boldsymbol{\Theta}$ becomes $\widehat{\boldsymbol{\Theta}}^B = (\boldsymbol{I}_m - \boldsymbol{\Omega})\boldsymbol{X}$. Since we need to estimate $\boldsymbol{\Omega}$, it will be estimated from the marginal distributions of $\boldsymbol{X}$ and $\boldsymbol{S}$. Then from Corollary 3.1, $E[\boldsymbol{X}\boldsymbol{\Sigma}^{-1}\boldsymbol{X}^\top] = p\boldsymbol{\Omega}^{-1}$, and we think of $\widehat{\boldsymbol{\Omega}} = c(\boldsymbol{X}\boldsymbol{S}^{-1}\boldsymbol{X}^\top)^{-1}$ as an estimator of $\boldsymbol{\Omega}$, where c is a positive constant. Thus the resulting Efron-Morris (1972) type empirical Bayes estimator of $\boldsymbol{\Theta}$ for $p \geq m$ can be expressed as

$$\widehat{\boldsymbol{\Theta}}_2^{EMK} = (\boldsymbol{I}_m - \widehat{\boldsymbol{\Omega}})\boldsymbol{X} = \{\boldsymbol{I}_m - c(\boldsymbol{X}\boldsymbol{S}^{-1}\boldsymbol{X}^\top)^{-1}\}\boldsymbol{X}.$$

The Efron-Morris type estimators given here have been studied by Konno (1991, 1992). For other empirical Bayes approaches, see Tsukuma and Kubokawa (2007).

6.2.2 The Unified Efron-Morris Type Estimator

Let us here give a unified form of empirical Bayes estimators $\widehat{\boldsymbol{\Theta}}_1^{EMK}$ and $\widehat{\boldsymbol{\Theta}}_2^{EMK}$ with properties of the Moore-Penrose inverse. When $m > p$ with $n \geq p$, using (i), (ii) and (iv) of Lemma 2.3 yields

$$(\boldsymbol{X}\boldsymbol{S}^{-1}\boldsymbol{X}^\top)^+ = (\boldsymbol{X}^\top)^+\boldsymbol{S}\boldsymbol{X}^+ = \boldsymbol{X}(\boldsymbol{X}^\top\boldsymbol{X})^{-1}\boldsymbol{S}(\boldsymbol{X}^\top\boldsymbol{X})^{-1}\boldsymbol{X}^\top,$$

so that $(\boldsymbol{X}\boldsymbol{S}^{-1}\boldsymbol{X}^\top)^+\boldsymbol{X} = \boldsymbol{X}(\boldsymbol{X}^\top\boldsymbol{X})^{-1}\boldsymbol{S}$. When $p \geq m$ with $n \geq p$, $\boldsymbol{X}\boldsymbol{S}^{-1}\boldsymbol{X}^\top$ is of full rank and its Moore-Penrose inverse becomes $(\boldsymbol{X}\boldsymbol{S}^{-1}\boldsymbol{X}^\top)^+ = (\boldsymbol{X}\boldsymbol{S}^{-1}\boldsymbol{X}^\top)^{-1}$. Hence for both cases of $m > p$ and $p \geq m$ with $n \geq p$, the Efron-Morris type empirical Bayes estimators $\widehat{\boldsymbol{\Theta}}_1^{EMK}$ and $\widehat{\boldsymbol{\Theta}}_2^{EMK}$ can be unified into $\widehat{\boldsymbol{\Theta}}^{EMK} = \boldsymbol{X} - c(\boldsymbol{X}\boldsymbol{S}^{-1}\boldsymbol{X}^\top)^+\boldsymbol{X}$, where c is a constant.

In the case of $p > n$, the rank of $\boldsymbol{S}$ is deficient and its inverse does not exist. Therefore, we replace $\boldsymbol{S}^{-1}$ with $\boldsymbol{S}^+$. This leads to $\widehat{\boldsymbol{\Theta}}^{EMK} = \boldsymbol{X} - c(\boldsymbol{X}\boldsymbol{S}^+\boldsymbol{X}^\top)^+\boldsymbol{X}$.

On the other hand, in the case where $m = 1$, Chételat and Wells (2012) suggested the shrinkage estimator

$$\widehat{\boldsymbol{\Theta}}^{CW} = \boldsymbol{X} - \frac{c}{\boldsymbol{X}\boldsymbol{S}^+\boldsymbol{X}^\top}\boldsymbol{X}\boldsymbol{S}\boldsymbol{S}^+.$$

An important problem is how to extend $\widehat{\boldsymbol{\Theta}}^{CW}$ to the framework of estimation of the mean matrix $\boldsymbol{\Theta}$. In particular, the Efron-Morris type estimator seems to take various variants which depend on possible orderings among m, n and p. One of interesting results provided here is that we can develop a unified form for the Efron-Morris type estimators, given by

$$\widehat{\boldsymbol{\Theta}}^{EMK} = \boldsymbol{X} - c(\boldsymbol{X}\boldsymbol{S}^+\boldsymbol{X}^\top)^+\boldsymbol{X}\boldsymbol{S}\boldsymbol{S}^+, \tag{6.9}$$

for any set of (m, n, p). Of course, the expression (6.9) includes $\widehat{\boldsymbol{\Theta}}_1^{EMK}$, $\widehat{\boldsymbol{\Theta}}_2^{EMK}$ and $\widehat{\boldsymbol{\Theta}}^{CW}$ as special cases.

The matrix $\boldsymbol{X}\boldsymbol{S}^+\boldsymbol{X}^\top$ is nonsingular for $n \wedge p \geq m$, while it is singular for $m > n \wedge p$. In fact, $(\boldsymbol{X}\boldsymbol{S}^+\boldsymbol{X}^\top)^+$ for $n \wedge p \geq m$ can be rewritten as

$$(\boldsymbol{X}\boldsymbol{S}^+\boldsymbol{X}^\top)^+ = \begin{cases} (\boldsymbol{X}\boldsymbol{S}^{-1}\boldsymbol{X}^\top)^{-1} & \text{for } n \geq p \geq m, \\ (\boldsymbol{X}\boldsymbol{S}^+\boldsymbol{X}^\top)^{-1} & \text{for } p > n \geq m, \end{cases}$$

and the corresponding Efron-Morris type estimators are provided. In the case of $m > n \wedge p$, $\widehat{\boldsymbol{\Theta}}^{EMK}$ in (6.9) can be expressed as in the following lemma.

Lemma 6.1 *In the case of $m > n \wedge p$, the Efron-Morris type estimators in (6.9) can be expressed as*

$$\widehat{\boldsymbol{\Theta}}^{EMK} = \begin{cases} \boldsymbol{X} - c\boldsymbol{X}(\boldsymbol{X}^\top\boldsymbol{X})^{-1}\boldsymbol{S} & \text{for } n \geq m > p \text{ or for } m > n \geq p, \\ \boldsymbol{X} - c\boldsymbol{X}(\boldsymbol{S}\boldsymbol{S}^+\boldsymbol{X}^\top\boldsymbol{X}\boldsymbol{S}\boldsymbol{S}^+)^+\boldsymbol{S} & \text{for } m > p > n \text{ or for } p \geq m > n. \end{cases} \tag{6.10}$$

Proof When $n \geq m > p$ or when $m > n \geq p$, using (i) of Lemma 2.3 gives $S^+ = S^{-1}$. Further from Lemma 2.3,

$$(XS^+X^\top)^+ \cdot XSS^+ = (X^\top)^+SX^+ \cdot X = X(X^\top X)^{-1}S,$$

which verifies the expression (6.10) when $n \geq m > p$ or when $m > n \geq p$.

When $m > p > n$ or when $p \geq m > n$, we denote the eigenvalue decomposition of S by $S = HLH^\top$, where $H \in \mathbb{V}_{p,n}$ and $L \in \mathbb{D}_n^{(\geq 0)}$. From (i) and (iv) of Lemma 2.3, $S^+ = HL^{-1}H^\top$, so that $SS^+ = HH^\top = S^+S$. Since XH $(\in \mathbb{R}^{m\times n})$ is of rank n, it is observed that

$$\begin{aligned}
(XS^+X^\top)^+XSS^+ &= (XHL^{-1}H^\top X^\top)^+XHH^\top \\
&= (H^\top X^\top)^+L(XH)^+XHH^\top && (\because \text{(iv) of Lemma 2.3}) \\
&= (H^\top X^\top)^+LH^\top && (\because \text{(iii) of Lemma 2.3}) \\
&= XH(H^\top X^\top XH)^{-1}LH^\top && (\because \text{(ii) of Lemma 2.3}) \\
&= XH(H^\top X^\top XH)^{-1}H^\top HLH^\top && (\because H^\top H = I_n) \\
&= XH(H^\top X^\top XH)^{-1}H^\top S && (\because S = HLH^\top).
\end{aligned}$$

Again from (i), (ii) and (iv) of Lemma 2.3,

$$H(H^\top X^\top XH)^{-1}H^\top = (HH^\top X^\top XHH^\top)^+ = (SS^+X^\top XSS^+)^+.$$

Hence the expression (6.10) is obtained for the case where $m > p > n$ or $p \geq m > n$. $\square$

6.3 A Unified Class of Matricial Shrinkage Estimators

To define the class (6.8), Konno (1992) separately considered two cases, where $m > p$ and where $p \geq m$, under $n \geq p$. The arguments stated in the previous section suggest that we can construct a well-defined class of matricial shrinkage estimators for all possible orders on m, n and p.

Hereafter in this chapter, we denote

$$\tau = m \wedge n \wedge p.$$

Define the eigenvalue decomposition of S as $S = HLH^\top$, where $H \in \mathbb{V}_{p,n\wedge p}$ and $L \in \mathbb{D}_{n\wedge p}^{(\geq 0)}$. Let $L^{1/2} = \operatorname{diag}(\sqrt{\ell_1}, \ldots, \sqrt{\ell_{n\wedge p}})$ and $L^{-1/2} = (L^{1/2})^{-1}$. Denote the singular value decomposition of $XHL^{-1/2}$ by

$$XHL^{-1/2} = RF^{1/2}V^\top,$$

where $\boldsymbol{R} \in \mathbb{V}_{m,\tau}$, $\boldsymbol{V} \in \mathbb{V}_{n\wedge p,\tau}$ and $\boldsymbol{F}^{1/2} = \mathrm{diag}\,(\sqrt{f_1}, \ldots, \sqrt{f_\tau}) \in \mathbb{D}_\tau^{(\geq 0)}$. It is clear that $\boldsymbol{X}\boldsymbol{S}^+\boldsymbol{X}^\top = \boldsymbol{X}\boldsymbol{H}\boldsymbol{L}^{-1}\boldsymbol{H}^\top\boldsymbol{X}^\top = \boldsymbol{R}\boldsymbol{F}\boldsymbol{R}^\top$, which is the eigenvalue decomposition of $\boldsymbol{X}\boldsymbol{S}^+\boldsymbol{X}^\top$. For any possible triplet (m, n, p), a unified class of matricial shrinkage estimators is defined by

$$\widehat{\boldsymbol{\Theta}}^{SH} = \widehat{\boldsymbol{\Theta}}^{SH}(\boldsymbol{X}, \boldsymbol{S}) = \boldsymbol{X} - \boldsymbol{R}\boldsymbol{\Phi}(\boldsymbol{F})\boldsymbol{R}^\top\boldsymbol{X}\boldsymbol{S}\boldsymbol{S}^+, \tag{6.11}$$

where $\boldsymbol{\Phi}(\boldsymbol{F}) = \mathrm{diag}\,(\phi_1(\boldsymbol{F}), \ldots, \phi_\tau(\boldsymbol{F})) \in \mathbb{D}_\tau$ and the $\phi_i(\boldsymbol{F})$'s are absolutely continuous functions of $\boldsymbol{F}$.

Let us here discuss invariance of the unified class (6.11) under the orthogonal transformations $\boldsymbol{X} \to \boldsymbol{O}\boldsymbol{X}\boldsymbol{P}$, $\boldsymbol{S} \to \boldsymbol{P}^\top\boldsymbol{S}\boldsymbol{P}$, $\boldsymbol{\Theta} \to \boldsymbol{O}\boldsymbol{\Theta}\boldsymbol{P}$ and $\boldsymbol{\Sigma} \to \boldsymbol{P}^\top\boldsymbol{\Sigma}\boldsymbol{P}$ for any $\boldsymbol{O} \in \mathbb{O}_m$ and $\boldsymbol{P} \in \mathbb{O}_p$. Then for an estimator $\widehat{\boldsymbol{\Theta}} = \widehat{\boldsymbol{\Theta}}(\boldsymbol{X}, \boldsymbol{S})$, it seems natural to require $\widehat{\boldsymbol{\Theta}}(\boldsymbol{O}\boldsymbol{X}\boldsymbol{P}, \boldsymbol{P}^\top\boldsymbol{S}\boldsymbol{P}) = \boldsymbol{O}\widehat{\boldsymbol{\Theta}}(\boldsymbol{X}, \boldsymbol{S})\boldsymbol{P}$. Since the eigenvalue decomposition of $\boldsymbol{P}^\top\boldsymbol{S}\boldsymbol{P}$ is $\boldsymbol{P}^\top\boldsymbol{H}\boldsymbol{L}\boldsymbol{H}^\top\boldsymbol{P}$, it turns out that, due to (i), (ii) and (iv) of Lemma 2.3,

$$\begin{aligned}(\boldsymbol{P}^\top\boldsymbol{S}\boldsymbol{P})^+ &= (\boldsymbol{H}^\top\boldsymbol{P})^+\boldsymbol{L}^{-1}(\boldsymbol{P}^\top\boldsymbol{H})^+ \\ &= \boldsymbol{P}^\top\boldsymbol{H}(\boldsymbol{H}^\top\boldsymbol{P}\boldsymbol{P}^\top\boldsymbol{H})^{-1}\boldsymbol{L}^{-1}(\boldsymbol{H}^\top\boldsymbol{P}\boldsymbol{P}^\top\boldsymbol{H})^{-1}\boldsymbol{H}^\top\boldsymbol{P} \\ &= \boldsymbol{P}^\top\boldsymbol{H}\boldsymbol{L}^{-1}\boldsymbol{H}^\top\boldsymbol{P} = \boldsymbol{P}^\top\boldsymbol{S}^+\boldsymbol{P}.\end{aligned}$$

Thus, $\boldsymbol{O}\boldsymbol{X}\boldsymbol{P}(\boldsymbol{P}^\top\boldsymbol{S}\boldsymbol{P})^+(\boldsymbol{O}\boldsymbol{X}\boldsymbol{P})^\top = \boldsymbol{O}\boldsymbol{X}\boldsymbol{S}^+\boldsymbol{X}^\top\boldsymbol{O}^\top$, whose eigenvalue decomposition is $\boldsymbol{O}\boldsymbol{R}\boldsymbol{F}\boldsymbol{R}^\top\boldsymbol{O}^\top$. This yields, for any $\boldsymbol{O} \in \mathbb{O}_m$ and $\boldsymbol{P} \in \mathbb{O}_p$,

$$\begin{aligned}\widehat{\boldsymbol{\Theta}}^{SH}(\boldsymbol{O}\boldsymbol{X}\boldsymbol{P}, \boldsymbol{P}^\top\boldsymbol{S}\boldsymbol{P}) &= \boldsymbol{O}\boldsymbol{X}\boldsymbol{P} - \boldsymbol{O}\boldsymbol{R}\cdot\boldsymbol{\Phi}(\boldsymbol{F})\cdot\boldsymbol{R}^\top\boldsymbol{O}^\top\cdot\boldsymbol{O}\boldsymbol{X}\boldsymbol{P}\cdot\boldsymbol{P}^\top\boldsymbol{S}\boldsymbol{P}\cdot(\boldsymbol{P}^\top\boldsymbol{S}\boldsymbol{P})^+ \\ &= \boldsymbol{O}\widehat{\boldsymbol{\Theta}}^{SH}(\boldsymbol{X}, \boldsymbol{S})\boldsymbol{P},\end{aligned}$$

which shows invariance of $\widehat{\boldsymbol{\Theta}}^{SH}$. Note that if $\boldsymbol{P} \in \mathbb{U}_p$ and $\boldsymbol{P} \notin \mathbb{O}_p$ with $p > n$ then $(\boldsymbol{P}^\top\boldsymbol{H})^+ \neq \boldsymbol{H}^\top\boldsymbol{P}$ and $\widehat{\boldsymbol{\Theta}}^{SH}$ does not retain invariance, namely, it is not invariant under the scale transformations (4.4).

The Efron-Morris type estimator (6.9) lies in the unified class (6.11). It indeed holds that, according to (i), (ii) and (iv) of Lemma 2.3, $(\boldsymbol{X}\boldsymbol{S}^+\boldsymbol{X}^\top)^+ = (\boldsymbol{R}\boldsymbol{F}\boldsymbol{R}^\top)^+ = \boldsymbol{R}\boldsymbol{F}^{-1}\boldsymbol{R}^\top$, yielding

$$\widehat{\boldsymbol{\Theta}}^{EMK} = \boldsymbol{X} - \boldsymbol{R}\boldsymbol{\Phi}^{EMK}(\boldsymbol{F})\boldsymbol{R}^\top\boldsymbol{X}\boldsymbol{S}\boldsymbol{S}^+, \quad \boldsymbol{\Phi}^{EMK}(\boldsymbol{F}) = c\boldsymbol{F}^{-1}. \tag{6.12}$$

Next, we give some convenient representations for (6.11).

Lemma 6.2 *The unified class in (6.11) can be rewritten by*

$$\widehat{\boldsymbol{\Theta}}^{SH} = \boldsymbol{X}(\boldsymbol{I}_p - \boldsymbol{S}\boldsymbol{S}^+) + \boldsymbol{R}\{\boldsymbol{I}_\tau - \boldsymbol{\Phi}(\boldsymbol{F})\}\boldsymbol{R}^\top\boldsymbol{X}\boldsymbol{S}\boldsymbol{S}^+.$$

Proof Since $\boldsymbol{S} = \boldsymbol{H}\boldsymbol{L}\boldsymbol{H}^\top$ and $\boldsymbol{X}\boldsymbol{H}\boldsymbol{L}^{-1/2} = \boldsymbol{R}\boldsymbol{F}^{1/2}\boldsymbol{V}^\top$ where $\boldsymbol{R} \in \mathbb{V}_{m,\tau}$, it is seen that

$$(\boldsymbol{I}_m - \boldsymbol{R}\boldsymbol{R}^\top)\boldsymbol{X}\boldsymbol{S}\boldsymbol{S}^+ = (\boldsymbol{I}_m - \boldsymbol{R}\boldsymbol{R}^\top)\boldsymbol{X}\boldsymbol{H}\boldsymbol{H}^\top$$
$$= (\boldsymbol{I}_m - \boldsymbol{R}\boldsymbol{R}^\top)\boldsymbol{R}\boldsymbol{F}^{1/2}\boldsymbol{V}^\top\boldsymbol{L}^{1/2}\boldsymbol{H}^\top = \boldsymbol{0}_{m\times p},$$

which is used to rewrite the class (6.11) as

$$\widehat{\boldsymbol{\Theta}}^{SH} = \boldsymbol{X} - \boldsymbol{X}\boldsymbol{S}\boldsymbol{S}^+ + \boldsymbol{X}\boldsymbol{S}\boldsymbol{S}^+ - \boldsymbol{R}\boldsymbol{R}^\top\boldsymbol{X}\boldsymbol{S}\boldsymbol{S}^+ + \boldsymbol{R}\boldsymbol{R}^\top\boldsymbol{X}\boldsymbol{S}\boldsymbol{S}^+ - \boldsymbol{R}\boldsymbol{\Phi}(\boldsymbol{F})\boldsymbol{R}^\top\boldsymbol{X}\boldsymbol{S}\boldsymbol{S}^+$$
$$= \boldsymbol{X}(\boldsymbol{I}_p - \boldsymbol{S}\boldsymbol{S}^+) + \boldsymbol{R}\{\boldsymbol{I}_\tau - \boldsymbol{\Phi}(\boldsymbol{F})\}\boldsymbol{R}^\top\boldsymbol{X}\boldsymbol{S}\boldsymbol{S}^+.$$

Hence the proof is complete. □

When $p > n$, because of (i), (ii) and (iv) in Lemma 2.3,

$$\boldsymbol{S}\boldsymbol{S}^+ = \boldsymbol{Y}^\top\boldsymbol{Y}\cdot(\boldsymbol{Y}^\top\boldsymbol{Y})^+ = \boldsymbol{Y}^\top\boldsymbol{Y}\cdot\boldsymbol{Y}^\top(\boldsymbol{Y}\boldsymbol{Y}^\top)^{-2}\boldsymbol{Y} = \boldsymbol{Y}^\top(\boldsymbol{Y}\boldsymbol{Y}^\top)^{-1}\boldsymbol{Y}$$

is the orthogonal projection matrix onto the subspace spanned by rows of $\boldsymbol{Y}$. The ML estimator is rewritten as $\widehat{\boldsymbol{\Theta}}^{ML} = \boldsymbol{X}(\boldsymbol{I}_p - \boldsymbol{S}\boldsymbol{S}^+) + \boldsymbol{X}\boldsymbol{S}\boldsymbol{S}^+$. Thus Lemma 6.2 implies that $\widehat{\boldsymbol{\Theta}}^{SH}$ is shrinking with respect only to the projections of rows of $\boldsymbol{X}$ onto the subspace spanned by rows of $\boldsymbol{Y}$.

Further, the unified class (6.11) can be rewritten as in the following lemma which is an extension for Konno's (1992) class (6.8) with $m > p$.

Lemma 6.3 *Let $\boldsymbol{Q} = \boldsymbol{H}\boldsymbol{L}^{-1/2}\boldsymbol{V} \in \mathbb{R}^{p\times\tau}$. Then $\boldsymbol{Q}^- = \boldsymbol{V}^\top\boldsymbol{L}^{1/2}\boldsymbol{H}^\top \in \mathbb{R}^{\tau\times p}$ is the generalized inverse of $\boldsymbol{Q}$. Further the unified class in (6.11) can be rewritten as*

$$\widehat{\boldsymbol{\Theta}}^{SH} = \boldsymbol{X}\{\boldsymbol{I}_p - \boldsymbol{Q}\boldsymbol{\Phi}(\boldsymbol{F})\boldsymbol{Q}^-\}$$
$$= \boldsymbol{X}(\boldsymbol{I}_p - \boldsymbol{S}\boldsymbol{S}^+) + \boldsymbol{X}\boldsymbol{S}\boldsymbol{S}^+\boldsymbol{Q}\{\boldsymbol{I}_\tau - \boldsymbol{\Phi}(\boldsymbol{F})\}\boldsymbol{Q}^-. \tag{6.13}$$

Proof It is seen that

$$\boldsymbol{Q}\boldsymbol{Q}^-\boldsymbol{Q} = \boldsymbol{H}\boldsymbol{L}^{-1/2}\boldsymbol{V}\boldsymbol{V}^\top\boldsymbol{L}^{1/2}\boldsymbol{H}^\top\boldsymbol{H}\boldsymbol{L}^{-1/2}\boldsymbol{V} = \boldsymbol{H}\boldsymbol{L}^{-1/2}\boldsymbol{V}\boldsymbol{V}^\top\boldsymbol{V} = \boldsymbol{H}\boldsymbol{L}^{-1/2}\boldsymbol{V} = \boldsymbol{Q},$$

and consequently $\boldsymbol{Q}^-$ is the generalized inverse of $\boldsymbol{Q}$. Since

$$\boldsymbol{R} = \boldsymbol{X}\boldsymbol{H}\boldsymbol{L}^{-1/2}\boldsymbol{V}\boldsymbol{F}^{-1/2} = \boldsymbol{X}\boldsymbol{Q}\boldsymbol{F}^{-1/2},$$
$$\boldsymbol{R}^\top\boldsymbol{X}\boldsymbol{S}\boldsymbol{S}^+ = \boldsymbol{R}^\top\boldsymbol{R}\boldsymbol{F}^{1/2}\boldsymbol{V}^\top\boldsymbol{L}^{1/2}\boldsymbol{H}^\top = \boldsymbol{F}^{1/2}\boldsymbol{Q}^-, \tag{6.14}$$

it follows that

$$\boldsymbol{R}\boldsymbol{\Phi}(\boldsymbol{F})\boldsymbol{R}^\top\boldsymbol{X}\boldsymbol{S}\boldsymbol{S}^+ = \boldsymbol{X}\boldsymbol{Q}\boldsymbol{F}^{-1/2}\boldsymbol{\Phi}(\boldsymbol{F})\boldsymbol{F}^{1/2}\boldsymbol{Q}^- = \boldsymbol{X}\boldsymbol{Q}\boldsymbol{\Phi}(\boldsymbol{F})\boldsymbol{Q}^-.$$

Hence, we get the first equality in (6.13). The second equality in (6.13) can be obtained similarly by using Lemma 6.2 with the fact that $\boldsymbol{Q} = \boldsymbol{S}\boldsymbol{S}^+\boldsymbol{Q}$. □

As for $\boldsymbol{Q}$ in Lemma 6.3, it is easy to check that $\boldsymbol{Q} = \boldsymbol{S}^{+}\boldsymbol{X}^{\top}\boldsymbol{R}\boldsymbol{F}^{-1/2}$ and $\boldsymbol{Q}^{-} = \boldsymbol{F}^{-1/2}\boldsymbol{R}^{\top}\boldsymbol{X}\boldsymbol{S}\boldsymbol{S}^{+}$. Also, $\boldsymbol{Q}^{\top}\boldsymbol{S}\boldsymbol{Q} = \boldsymbol{I}_{\tau}$ and $\boldsymbol{Q}^{\top}\boldsymbol{X}^{\top}\boldsymbol{X}\boldsymbol{Q} = \boldsymbol{F}$, while

$$(\boldsymbol{Q}^{-})^{\top}\boldsymbol{Q}^{-} = \begin{cases} \boldsymbol{S} & \text{for } m > n \wedge p, \\ \boldsymbol{S}\boldsymbol{S}^{+}\boldsymbol{X}^{\top}(\boldsymbol{X}\boldsymbol{S}^{+}\boldsymbol{X}^{\top})^{-1}\boldsymbol{X}\boldsymbol{S}\boldsymbol{S}^{+} & \text{for } m \le n \wedge p, \end{cases}$$

and

$$(\boldsymbol{Q}^{-})^{\top}\boldsymbol{F}\boldsymbol{Q}^{-} = \begin{cases} \boldsymbol{X}^{\top}\boldsymbol{X} & \text{for } n \ge p \ge m, \\ \boldsymbol{S}\boldsymbol{S}^{+}\boldsymbol{X}^{\top}(\boldsymbol{X}\boldsymbol{S}^{+}\boldsymbol{X}^{\top})(\boldsymbol{X}\boldsymbol{S}^{+}\boldsymbol{X}^{\top})^{+}\boldsymbol{X}\boldsymbol{S}\boldsymbol{S}^{+} & \text{otherwise.} \end{cases}$$

Lemmas 6.2 and 6.3 suggest that $\widehat{\boldsymbol{\Theta}}^{SH}$ shrinks not only columns, but also rows of $\boldsymbol{X}\boldsymbol{S}\boldsymbol{S}^{+}$ in terms of $\widehat{\boldsymbol{\Theta}}^{ML}$.

If all the diagonals of $\boldsymbol{\Phi}(\boldsymbol{F})$ are positive and the matrix square root of $\boldsymbol{\Phi}(\boldsymbol{F})$ is denoted by $\boldsymbol{\Phi}^{1/2}$ then

$$\boldsymbol{R}\boldsymbol{\Phi}\boldsymbol{F}\boldsymbol{R}^{\top}\boldsymbol{X}\boldsymbol{S}\boldsymbol{S}^{+} = \boldsymbol{R}\boldsymbol{\Phi}^{1/2}\boldsymbol{R}^{\top}\boldsymbol{R}\boldsymbol{\Phi}^{1/2}\boldsymbol{R}^{\top}\boldsymbol{X}\boldsymbol{S}\boldsymbol{S}^{+} = \boldsymbol{R}\boldsymbol{\Phi}^{1/2}\boldsymbol{R}^{\top}\boldsymbol{X}\boldsymbol{Q}\boldsymbol{\Phi}^{1/2}\boldsymbol{Q}^{-}.$$

Since $\boldsymbol{Q} = \boldsymbol{S}\boldsymbol{S}^{+}\boldsymbol{Q}$, we get the following lemma as well.

Lemma 6.4 *If all the diagonals of $\boldsymbol{\Phi}(\boldsymbol{F})$ are positive and the matrix square root of $\boldsymbol{\Phi}(\boldsymbol{F})$ is denoted by $\boldsymbol{\Phi}^{1/2}$ then the unified class (6.11) can be rewritten by*

$$\widehat{\boldsymbol{\Theta}}^{SH} = \boldsymbol{X} - \boldsymbol{R}\boldsymbol{\Phi}^{1/2}\boldsymbol{R}^{\top}\boldsymbol{X}\boldsymbol{S}\boldsymbol{S}^{+}\boldsymbol{Q}\boldsymbol{\Phi}^{1/2}\boldsymbol{Q}^{-}.$$

If all the diagonals of $\boldsymbol{I}_{\tau} - \boldsymbol{\Phi}(\boldsymbol{F})$ are positive and the matrix square root of $\boldsymbol{I}_{\tau} - \boldsymbol{\Phi}(\boldsymbol{F})$ is denoted by $(\boldsymbol{I}_{\tau} - \boldsymbol{\Phi})^{1/2}$ then the unified class (6.11) can be rewritten by

$$\widehat{\boldsymbol{\Theta}}^{SH} = \boldsymbol{X}(\boldsymbol{I}_{p} - \boldsymbol{S}\boldsymbol{S}^{+}) + \boldsymbol{R}(\boldsymbol{I}_{\tau} - \boldsymbol{\Phi})^{1/2}\boldsymbol{R}^{\top}\boldsymbol{X}\boldsymbol{S}\boldsymbol{S}^{+}\boldsymbol{Q}(\boldsymbol{I}_{\tau} - \boldsymbol{\Phi})^{1/2}\boldsymbol{Q}^{-}.$$

As seen in the above lemmas, $\widehat{\boldsymbol{\Theta}}^{SH}$ takes several different forms. In the following, we will employ the different forms for different purposes.

6.4 Unbiased Risk Estimate

Abbreviate $\boldsymbol{\Phi}(\boldsymbol{F})$ to $\boldsymbol{\Phi}$. The quadratic loss (6.7) of $\widehat{\boldsymbol{\Theta}}^{SH}$ in (6.11) is expanded to

$$\begin{aligned} L(\widehat{\boldsymbol{\Theta}}^{SH}, \boldsymbol{\Theta}|\boldsymbol{\Sigma}) = {} & \operatorname{tr}(\boldsymbol{X} - \boldsymbol{\Theta})\boldsymbol{\Sigma}^{-1}(\boldsymbol{X} - \boldsymbol{\Theta})^{\top} - 2\operatorname{tr}(\boldsymbol{X} - \boldsymbol{\Theta})\boldsymbol{\Sigma}^{-1}\boldsymbol{S}\boldsymbol{S}^{+}\boldsymbol{X}^{\top}\boldsymbol{R}\boldsymbol{\Phi}\boldsymbol{R}^{\top} \\ & + \operatorname{tr}\boldsymbol{R}\boldsymbol{\Phi}\boldsymbol{R}^{\top}\boldsymbol{X}\boldsymbol{S}\boldsymbol{S}^{+}\boldsymbol{\Sigma}^{-1}\boldsymbol{S}\boldsymbol{S}^{+}\boldsymbol{X}^{\top}\boldsymbol{R}\boldsymbol{\Phi}\boldsymbol{R}^{\top}. \end{aligned}$$

Recalling that $R(\boldsymbol{X}, \boldsymbol{\Theta}) = mp$, we obtain $R(\widehat{\boldsymbol{\Theta}}^{SH}, \boldsymbol{\Theta}) = mp + E_2 - 2E_1$, where

$$E_1 = E[\operatorname{tr}(\boldsymbol{X} - \boldsymbol{\Theta})\boldsymbol{\Sigma}^{-1}\boldsymbol{S}\boldsymbol{S}^{+}\boldsymbol{X}^{\top}\boldsymbol{R}\boldsymbol{\Phi}\boldsymbol{R}^{\top}], \quad E_2 = E[\operatorname{tr}\boldsymbol{\Sigma}^{-1}\boldsymbol{S}\boldsymbol{S}^{+}\boldsymbol{X}^{\top}\boldsymbol{R}\boldsymbol{\Phi}^{2}\boldsymbol{R}^{\top}\boldsymbol{X}\boldsymbol{S}\boldsymbol{S}^{+}].$$

Here Theorem 5.1, or (5.3), is used to evaluate E_1. If the conditions in Theorem 5.1 are satisfied for $\boldsymbol{G}_1 = \boldsymbol{I}_m$ and $\boldsymbol{G}_2 = \boldsymbol{\Sigma}^{-1}\boldsymbol{S}\boldsymbol{S}^{+}\boldsymbol{X}^{\top}\boldsymbol{R}\boldsymbol{\Phi}\boldsymbol{R}^{\top}$, then E_1 can be expressed as

$$E_1 = E[\,\mathrm{tr}\,\nabla_X \boldsymbol{S}\boldsymbol{S}^{+}\boldsymbol{X}^{\top}\boldsymbol{R}\boldsymbol{\Phi}\boldsymbol{R}^{\top}].$$

Similarly, since $\boldsymbol{Y} \sim \mathcal{N}_{n\times p}(\boldsymbol{0}_{n\times p}, \boldsymbol{I}_n \otimes \boldsymbol{\Sigma})$, Theorem 5.1 is used to rewrite E_2 as

$$\begin{aligned} E_2 &= E[\,\mathrm{tr}\,\boldsymbol{\Sigma}^{-1}\boldsymbol{Y}^{\top}\boldsymbol{Y}\boldsymbol{S}^{+}\boldsymbol{X}^{\top}\boldsymbol{R}\boldsymbol{\Phi}^2\boldsymbol{R}^{\top}\boldsymbol{X}\boldsymbol{S}\boldsymbol{S}^{+}] \\ &= E[\,\mathrm{tr}\,\nabla_Y^{\top}\boldsymbol{Y}\boldsymbol{S}^{+}\boldsymbol{X}^{\top}\boldsymbol{R}\boldsymbol{\Phi}^2\boldsymbol{R}^{\top}\boldsymbol{X}\boldsymbol{S}\boldsymbol{S}^{+}]. \end{aligned}$$

A sufficient condition for applying Theorem 5.1 to E_1 and E_2 is

$$E[\,\mathrm{tr}\,\boldsymbol{S}\cdot\,\mathrm{tr}\,\boldsymbol{F}\boldsymbol{\Phi}^2] < \infty. \tag{6.15}$$

For more details, see Tsukuma and Kubokawa (2015).

From the above observation, an unbiased risk estimate of $\widehat{\boldsymbol{\Theta}}^{SH}$ is given by

$$\widehat{R}(\widehat{\boldsymbol{\Theta}}^{SH}) = mp + \,\mathrm{tr}\,\nabla_Y^{\top}\boldsymbol{Y}\boldsymbol{S}^{+}\boldsymbol{X}^{\top}\boldsymbol{R}\boldsymbol{\Phi}^2\boldsymbol{R}^{\top}\boldsymbol{X}\boldsymbol{S}\boldsymbol{S}^{+} - 2\,\mathrm{tr}\,\nabla_X\boldsymbol{S}\boldsymbol{S}^{+}\boldsymbol{X}^{\top}\boldsymbol{R}\boldsymbol{\Phi}\boldsymbol{R}^{\top}.$$

Using Lemmas 6.6 and 6.7 in the Appendix yields

Theorem 6.1 *Let $\phi_i = \phi_i(\boldsymbol{F})$ for $i = 1, \ldots, \tau$. Assume that (6.15) is satisfied. For any possible ordering on m, n and p, an unbiased risk estimate of $\widehat{\boldsymbol{\Theta}}^{SH}$ is*

$$\begin{aligned} \widehat{R}(\widehat{\boldsymbol{\Theta}}^{SH}) = mp + \sum_{i=1}^{\tau}\Bigg\{ & a f_i\phi_i^2 - 2b\phi_i - 4f_i^2\phi_i\frac{\partial\phi_i}{\partial f_i} - 4f_i\frac{\partial\phi_i}{\partial f_i} \\ & - 2\sum_{j>i}^{\tau}\frac{f_i^2\phi_i^2 - f_j^2\phi_j^2}{f_i - f_j} - 4\sum_{j>i}^{\tau}\frac{f_i\phi_i - f_j\phi_j}{f_i - f_j}\Bigg\}, \end{aligned}$$

where $a = a_{m,p,n} = (|n-p| + 2m)\wedge(n+p) - 3$ and $b = b_{m,p,n} = |n\wedge p - m| + 1$.

The unbiased risk estimate $\widehat{R}(\widehat{\boldsymbol{\Theta}}^{SH})$ in Theorem 6.1 depends on $\boldsymbol{F} \in \mathbb{D}_{\tau}^{(\geq 0)}$. Let $\widehat{\boldsymbol{\Theta}}_0^{SH}$ and $\widehat{\boldsymbol{\Theta}}_1^{SH}$ be estimators belonging to the unified class (6.11). If $\widehat{R}(\widehat{\boldsymbol{\Theta}}_0^{SH}) \leq \widehat{R}(\widehat{\boldsymbol{\Theta}}_1^{SH})$ for any $\boldsymbol{F} \in \mathbb{D}_{\tau}^{(\geq 0)}$ and fixed (m, n, p), then $\widehat{\boldsymbol{\Theta}}_0^{SH}$ dominates $\widehat{\boldsymbol{\Theta}}_1^{SH}$ relative to the quadratic loss (6.7). For example, we have

Corollary 6.1 *If $\widehat{R}(\widehat{\boldsymbol{\Theta}}^{SH}) \leq \widehat{R}(\widehat{\boldsymbol{\Theta}}^{ML}) = mp$ for any $\boldsymbol{F} \in \mathbb{D}_{\tau}^{(\geq 0)}$ and fixed (m, n, p) then $\widehat{\boldsymbol{\Theta}}^{SH}$ is a minimax estimator dominating $\widehat{\boldsymbol{\Theta}}^{ML}$ relative to the quadratic loss (6.7).*

6.5 Examples for Specific Estimators

6.5.1 The Unified Efron-Morris Type Estimator

The unified Efron-Morris type estimator $\widehat{\boldsymbol{\Theta}}^{EMK}$ could be rewritten as in (6.12). To apply Theorem 6.1 to $\widehat{\boldsymbol{\Theta}}^{EMK}$, we put $\phi_i = cf_i^{-1}$. Then condition (6.15) is expressed by $c^2 E[\operatorname{tr} \boldsymbol{S} \operatorname{tr} \boldsymbol{F}^{-1}] < \infty$, which is satisfied if $b \geq 3$ or, equivalently, $|n \wedge p - m| \geq 2$ (see Lemma 6.8 of Tsukuma and Kubokawa 2015). The unbiased risk estimate of $\widehat{\boldsymbol{\Theta}}^{EMK}$ is

$$\widehat{R}(\widehat{\boldsymbol{\Theta}}^{EMK}) = mp + \{(a+4)c - 2(b-2)\}c \sum_{i=1}^{\tau} \frac{1}{f_i},$$

implying that if $0 < c \leq 2(b-2)/(a+4)$ and $b \geq 3$ then $\widehat{\boldsymbol{\Theta}}^{EMK}$ dominates $\widehat{\boldsymbol{\Theta}}^{ML}$ relative to the quadratic loss (6.7).

The unbiased risk estimate $\widehat{R}(\widehat{\boldsymbol{\Theta}}^{EMK})$ is a quadratic function of c and attains its minimum at

$$c^{EM} = \frac{b-2}{a+4} = \frac{|n \wedge p - m| - 1}{(|n-p| + 2m) \wedge (n+p) + 1}. \tag{6.16}$$

Define

$$\widehat{\boldsymbol{\Theta}}^{EM} = \boldsymbol{X} - c^{EM} \boldsymbol{R}\boldsymbol{F}^{-1}\boldsymbol{R}^{\top}\boldsymbol{X}\boldsymbol{S}\boldsymbol{S}^{+} = \boldsymbol{X} - c^{EM}(\boldsymbol{X}\boldsymbol{S}^{+}\boldsymbol{X}^{\top})^{+}\boldsymbol{X}\boldsymbol{S}\boldsymbol{S}^{+}. \tag{6.17}$$

This is an extension of Efron and Morris' (1972) original estimator in (6.1). The unbiased risk estimate of $\widehat{\boldsymbol{\Theta}}^{EM}$ has the form

$$\widehat{R}(\widehat{\boldsymbol{\Theta}}^{EM}) = mp - (b-2)c^{EM} \sum_{i=1}^{\tau} \frac{1}{f_i} = \widehat{R}(\widehat{\boldsymbol{\Theta}}^{ML}) - (b-2)c^{EM} \operatorname{tr} \boldsymbol{F}^{-1}. \tag{6.18}$$

When m, n and p are given, the corresponding specific values of a and b in c^{EM} are determined. Noting that $(|n-p| + 2m) \wedge (n+p) = n+p$ for $m > n \wedge p$, we can obtain specific values of c^{EM},

$$c^{EM} = \begin{cases} (p-m-1)/(n-p+2m+1) & \text{for } n \geq p \geq m, \\ (n-m-1)/(p-n+2m+1) & \text{for } p > n \geq m, \\ (m-p-1)/(n+p+1) & \text{for } n \geq m > p \text{ and } m > n \geq p, \\ (m-n-1)/(n+p+1) & \text{for } m > p > n \text{ and } p \geq m > n. \end{cases}$$

The cases satisfying $n \geq p$, namely, $n \geq p \geq m$, $n \geq m > p$ and $m > n \geq p$, are provided by Konno (1992).

6.5.2 A Modified Stein-Type Estimator

A modified Stein-type estimator is defined by

$$\widehat{\boldsymbol{\Theta}}^{mST} = \widehat{\boldsymbol{\Theta}}^{ST} - \frac{d}{\operatorname{tr} \boldsymbol{X}\boldsymbol{S}^{+}\boldsymbol{X}^{\top}} \boldsymbol{R}\boldsymbol{R}^{\top}\boldsymbol{X}\boldsymbol{S}\boldsymbol{S}^{+},$$

where $\widehat{\boldsymbol{\Theta}}^{ST} = \boldsymbol{X} - \boldsymbol{R}\boldsymbol{C}\boldsymbol{F}^{-1}\boldsymbol{R}^{\top}\boldsymbol{X}\boldsymbol{S}\boldsymbol{S}^{+}$ for $\boldsymbol{C} = \operatorname{diag}(c_1, \ldots, c_\tau)$ with $c_1 \geq \cdots \geq c_\tau$. This corresponds to the form

$$\phi_i = \frac{c_i}{f_i} + \frac{d}{\sum_{j=1}^{\tau} f_j} = \frac{c_i}{f_i} + \frac{d}{\operatorname{tr} \boldsymbol{F}}.$$

Then, from Theorem 6.1, it follows that

$$\begin{aligned}
\widehat{\Delta} &= \widehat{R}(\widehat{\boldsymbol{\Theta}}^{mST}) - \widehat{R}(\widehat{\boldsymbol{\Theta}}^{ML}) \\
&= \sum_{i=1}^{\tau} \frac{1}{f_i}(ac_i^2 - 2bc_i + 4c_i + 4c_i^2) \\
&\quad + \frac{1}{\operatorname{tr} \boldsymbol{F}} \left\{ (a - 2\tau + 2)d^2 - 2\tau bd - 2\tau(\tau - 1)d + 4d + 2(a + 2)d \sum_{i=1}^{\tau} c_i \right\} \\
&\quad + 4d \frac{\operatorname{tr} \boldsymbol{C}\boldsymbol{F}}{(\operatorname{tr} \boldsymbol{F})^2} + 4d^2 \frac{\operatorname{tr} \boldsymbol{F}^2}{(\operatorname{tr} \boldsymbol{F})^3} - 2 \sum_{i=1}^{\tau} \sum_{j>i}^{\tau} \frac{(c_i - c_j)(c_i + c_j + 2)}{f_i - f_j} \\
&\quad - \frac{4d}{\operatorname{tr} \boldsymbol{F}} \sum_{i=1}^{\tau} \sum_{j>i}^{\tau} \frac{c_i f_i - c_j f_j}{f_i - f_j},
\end{aligned} \tag{6.19}$$

because $\sum_{i=1}^{\tau} \sum_{j>i}^{\tau} (f_i + f_j) = (\tau - 1) \operatorname{tr} \boldsymbol{F}$. The condition for obtaining (6.19), namely, for satisfying (6.15), is $b \geq 3$. It is noted that $\operatorname{tr} \boldsymbol{F}^2 \leq (\operatorname{tr} \boldsymbol{F})^2$, $\operatorname{tr} \boldsymbol{C}\boldsymbol{F}/(\operatorname{tr} \boldsymbol{F})^2 \leq c_1/\operatorname{tr} \boldsymbol{F}$,

$$\sum_{i=1}^{\tau} \sum_{j>i}^{\tau} \frac{(c_i - c_j)(c_i + c_j + 2)}{f_i - f_j} \geq \sum_{i=1}^{\tau} \frac{1}{f_i} \sum_{j>i}^{\tau} (c_i - c_j)(c_i + c_j + 2),$$

$$\sum_{i=1}^{\tau} \sum_{j>i}^{\tau} \frac{c_i f_i - c_j f_j}{f_i - f_j} \geq \sum_{i=1}^{\tau} (\tau - i)c_i.$$

Thus, $\widehat{\Delta} \leq \sum_{i=1}^{\tau} h_c(i)/f_i + h_d/\operatorname{tr} \boldsymbol{F}$, where

$$h_c(i) = (a+4-2\tau+2i)c_i^2 - 2(b-2+2\tau-2i)c_i + 2\sum_{j>i}^{\tau} c_j(c_j+2),$$

$$h_d = (a-2\tau+6)d^2 - 2\left\{b\tau + \tau(\tau-1) - 2 - 2c_1 - (a+2)\sum_{i=1}^{\tau} c_i + 2\sum_{i=1}^{\tau}(\tau-i)c_i\right\}d.$$

For $i = 1, \ldots, \tau$, put

$$c_i = \frac{b-2+2\tau-2i}{a+4-2\tau+2i}, \tag{6.20}$$

which satisfy $c_1 \ge \cdots \ge c_\tau$ and $c_\tau = c^{EM}$ given in (6.16). Since $h_c(i)$ is a quadratic function of c_i, and $(a+4-2\tau+2i)c_i^2 - 2(b-2+2\tau-2i)c_i \le (a+4-2\tau+2i)c_{i+1}^2 - 2(b-2+2\tau-2i)c_{i+1}$ for each i, it is observed that

$$\begin{aligned}
h_c(i) &= (a+4-2\tau+2i)c_i^2 - 2(b-2+2\tau-2i)c_i + 2c_{i+1}(c_{i+1}+2) + 2\sum_{j>i+1}^{\tau} c_j(c_j+2) \\
&\le \{a+4-2\tau+2(i+1)\}c_{i+1}^2 - 2\{b-2+2\tau-2(i+1)\}c_{i+1} + 2\sum_{j>i+1}^{\tau} c_j(c_j+2) \\
&\le \cdots \le (a+2)c_{\tau-1}^2 - 2bc_{\tau-1} + 2c_\tau(c_\tau+2) \le (a+4)c_\tau^2 - 2(b-2)c_\tau \\
&= -(b-2)c_\tau = -(b-2)c^{EM}.
\end{aligned}$$

It is also seen that $2\sum_{i=1}^{\tau}(\tau-i)c_i = -(b+\tau-3)\tau + (a+4)\sum_{i=1}^{\tau} c_i$, which provides

$$h_d = (a-2\tau+6)d^2 - 4\left(\tau - 1 + \sum_{i=2}^{\tau} c_i\right)d.$$

Hence, from (6.18),

$$\widehat{\Delta} \le \widehat{R}(\widehat{\mathbf{\Theta}}^{EM}) - \widehat{R}(\widehat{\mathbf{\Theta}}^{ML}) + \left\{(a-2\tau+6)d^2 - 4\left(\tau - 1 + \sum_{i=2}^{\tau} c_i\right)d\right\}\frac{1}{\operatorname{tr} \boldsymbol{F}}.$$

These observations imply that $\widehat{\mathbf{\Theta}}^{ML}$ and $\widehat{\mathbf{\Theta}}^{EM}$ are improved on by $\widehat{\mathbf{\Theta}}^{ST} = \boldsymbol{X} - \boldsymbol{R}\boldsymbol{C}\boldsymbol{F}^{-1}\boldsymbol{R}^\top\boldsymbol{X}\boldsymbol{S}\boldsymbol{S}^+$ with constants c_i's given in (6.20). With these c_i's, $\widehat{\mathbf{\Theta}}^{ST}$ is an extension of Stein's (1973) estimator in (6.5) and further improved on by the modified Stein-type estimator

$$\widehat{\mathbf{\Theta}}^{mST} = \boldsymbol{X} - \boldsymbol{R}\boldsymbol{C}\boldsymbol{F}^{-1}\boldsymbol{R}^\top\boldsymbol{X}\boldsymbol{S}\boldsymbol{S}^+ - \frac{d}{\operatorname{tr}\boldsymbol{X}\boldsymbol{S}^+\boldsymbol{X}^\top}\boldsymbol{R}\boldsymbol{R}^\top\boldsymbol{X}\boldsymbol{S}\boldsymbol{S}^+$$

if d satisfies $0 < d \le 4\{\tau - 1 + \sum_{i=2}^{\tau} c_i\}/(a-2\tau+6)$. This is a generalization of Tsukuma and Kubokawa (2007) for any possible ordering on m, n and p.

6.5.3 Modified Efron-Morris Type Estimator

Next, we extend the modified Efron-Morris (1976) estimator in (6.3) to the unknown covariance case. Let

$$\widehat{\boldsymbol{\Theta}}^{mEM} = \widehat{\boldsymbol{\Theta}}^{EM} - \frac{d}{\operatorname{tr} \boldsymbol{X}\boldsymbol{S}^{+}\boldsymbol{X}^{\top}} \boldsymbol{R}\boldsymbol{R}^{\top}\boldsymbol{X}\boldsymbol{S}\boldsymbol{S}^{+},$$

where $\widehat{\boldsymbol{\Theta}}^{EM}$ is given in (6.17). This corresponds to the form

$$\phi_i = \frac{c^{EM}}{f_i} + \frac{d}{\sum_{j=1}^{\tau} f_j} = \frac{c^{EM}}{f_i} + \frac{d}{\operatorname{tr} \boldsymbol{F}}.$$

Letting $c_i = c^{EM}$ in (6.19) for all i and using the fact that $\operatorname{tr} \boldsymbol{F}^2 \le (\operatorname{tr} \boldsymbol{F})^2$, we get

$$\begin{aligned}
&\widehat{R}(\widehat{\boldsymbol{\Theta}}^{mEM}) - \widehat{R}(\widehat{\boldsymbol{\Theta}}^{ML}) \\
&\le -(b-2)c^{EM} \operatorname{tr} \boldsymbol{F}^{-1} \\
&\quad + \left\{(a-2\tau+2)d^2 - 2\tau b d - 2\tau(\tau-1)d + 4d + 2\tau(a+2)c^{EM} d\right\} \frac{1}{\operatorname{tr} \boldsymbol{F}} \\
&\quad + \frac{4c^{EM} d}{\operatorname{tr} \boldsymbol{F}} + \frac{4d^2}{\operatorname{tr} \boldsymbol{F}} - \frac{4c^{EM} d}{\operatorname{tr} \boldsymbol{F}} \sum_{i=1}^{\tau} (\tau - i).
\end{aligned}$$

With some algebraic manipulation,

$$\widehat{R}(\widehat{\boldsymbol{\Theta}}^{mEM}) - \widehat{R}(\widehat{\boldsymbol{\Theta}}^{EM}) \le \left[(a-2\tau+6)d^2 - 2d\frac{(a+b+2)(\tau-1)(\tau+2)}{a+4}\right] \frac{1}{\operatorname{tr} \boldsymbol{F}}. \tag{6.21}$$

Therefore $\widehat{\boldsymbol{\Theta}}^{mEM}$ improves on $\widehat{\boldsymbol{\Theta}}^{EM}$ if

$$0 < d \le 2\frac{(a+b+2)(\tau-1)(\tau+2)}{(a+4)(a-2\tau+6)}$$

for $b \ge 3$ and $\tau \ge 2$. The r.h.s. of (6.21) is quadratic in d and attains its minimum at

$$d_0 = \frac{(a+b+2)(\tau-1)(\tau+2)}{(a+4)(a-2\tau+6)} = \frac{(m+n\vee p)(m\wedge n\wedge p-1)(m\wedge n\wedge p+2)}{\{(|n-p|+2m)\wedge(n+p)+1\}(|n-p|+3)}.$$

That is, the Efron-Morris type estimator $\widehat{\boldsymbol{\Theta}}^{EM}$ is dominated by the modified Efron-Morris type estimator

$$\widehat{\boldsymbol{\Theta}}^{mEM} = \widehat{\boldsymbol{\Theta}}^{EM} - \frac{d_0}{\operatorname{tr} \boldsymbol{X}\boldsymbol{S}^+\boldsymbol{X}^\top}\boldsymbol{R}\boldsymbol{R}^\top\boldsymbol{X}\boldsymbol{S}\boldsymbol{S}^+$$

for $b \geq 3$ and $\tau \geq 2$.

6.6 Related Topics

6.6.1 Positive-Part Rule Estimators

In the field of estimating a mean vector of the multivariate normal distribution, a positive-part rule for shrinkage estimators is well known as an improving method of risk. For an analytical proof of the improvement, see Baranchik (1970). Gruber (1998) provided in detail numerical examples to compare risk performance of the James-Stein (1961) shrinkage and the corresponding positive-part rule estimators. In this section, we will give a positive-part rule for matricial shrinkage estimator (6.11).

With the help of Lemma 6.2, denote

$$\widehat{\boldsymbol{\Theta}}^{SH} = \boldsymbol{X}(\boldsymbol{I}_p - \boldsymbol{S}\boldsymbol{S}^+) + \boldsymbol{R}\boldsymbol{\Psi}(\boldsymbol{F})\boldsymbol{R}^\top\boldsymbol{X}\boldsymbol{S}\boldsymbol{S}^+,$$

where $\boldsymbol{\Psi}(\boldsymbol{F}) = \operatorname{diag}(\psi_1(\boldsymbol{F}), \dots, \psi_\tau(\boldsymbol{F})) = \boldsymbol{I}_\tau - \boldsymbol{\Phi}(\boldsymbol{F})$. Instead of $\boldsymbol{\Psi}(\boldsymbol{F})$, we here use $\boldsymbol{\Psi}_+(\boldsymbol{F}) = \operatorname{diag}(\psi_1^+(\boldsymbol{F}), \dots, \psi_\tau^+(\boldsymbol{F}))$ for $\psi_i^+(\boldsymbol{F}) = \max\{0, \psi_i(\boldsymbol{F})\}$. The resulting estimator is denoted by

$$\widehat{\boldsymbol{\Theta}}_+^{SH} = \boldsymbol{X}(\boldsymbol{I}_p - \boldsymbol{S}\boldsymbol{S}^+) + \boldsymbol{R}\boldsymbol{\Psi}_+(\boldsymbol{F})\boldsymbol{R}^\top\boldsymbol{X}\boldsymbol{S}\boldsymbol{S}^+.$$

If $m = 1$ with $n \geq p$, then $\widehat{\boldsymbol{\Theta}}_+^{SH}$ is the same as Baranchik's (1970) positive-part rule estimator. An analytical dominance result for $m > 1$ with $n \geq p$ was given by Tsukuma (2010). When $m = 1$ with $p > n$, $\widehat{\boldsymbol{\Theta}}_+^{SH}$ was suggested by Chételat and Wells (2012), who showed by simulation that $\widehat{\boldsymbol{\Theta}}_+^{SH}$ outperforms $\widehat{\boldsymbol{\Theta}}^{SH}$. These kind of dominance results can be proved unifiedly for any set (m, n, p).

Theorem 6.2 *Assume that* $\Pr(\psi_i(\boldsymbol{F}) < 0) > 0$ *for some* i. *Then* $\widehat{\boldsymbol{\Theta}}_+^{SH}$ *dominates* $\widehat{\boldsymbol{\Theta}}^{SH}$ *relative to the quadratic loss* (6.7) *regardless of an order relation among* m, n *and* p.

Proof Abbreviate $\boldsymbol{\Psi}(\boldsymbol{F}) = \operatorname{diag}(\psi_1(\boldsymbol{F}), \dots, \psi_\tau(\boldsymbol{F}))$ to $\boldsymbol{\Psi} = \operatorname{diag}(\psi_1, \dots, \psi_\tau)$ and $\boldsymbol{\Psi}_+(\boldsymbol{F}) = \operatorname{diag}(\psi_1^+(\boldsymbol{F}), \dots, \psi_\tau^+(\boldsymbol{F}))$ to $\boldsymbol{\Psi}_+ = \operatorname{diag}(\psi_1^+, \dots, \psi_\tau^+)$, respectively. Put $\nu = n \wedge p$. Let $\boldsymbol{H}_0 \in \mathbb{R}^{p\times(p-\nu)}$ such that $(\boldsymbol{H}, \boldsymbol{H}_0) \in \mathbb{O}_p$. We can express $\widehat{\boldsymbol{\Theta}}^{SH}$ as $\widehat{\boldsymbol{\Theta}}^{SH} = \boldsymbol{X}\boldsymbol{H}_0\boldsymbol{H}_0^\top + \boldsymbol{R}\boldsymbol{\Psi}\boldsymbol{R}^\top\boldsymbol{X}\boldsymbol{H}\boldsymbol{H}^\top$. Note that

$$\begin{aligned}\operatorname{tr}(\widehat{\boldsymbol{\Theta}}^{SH}-\boldsymbol{\Theta})\boldsymbol{\Sigma}^{-1}(\widehat{\boldsymbol{\Theta}}^{SH}-\boldsymbol{\Theta})^\top &= \operatorname{tr}(\boldsymbol{X}\boldsymbol{H}_0\boldsymbol{H}_0^\top-\boldsymbol{\Theta})\boldsymbol{\Sigma}^{-1}(\boldsymbol{X}\boldsymbol{H}_0\boldsymbol{H}_0^\top-\boldsymbol{\Theta})^\top\\ &\quad+2\operatorname{tr}\boldsymbol{\Psi}\boldsymbol{R}^\top\boldsymbol{X}\boldsymbol{H}\boldsymbol{H}^\top\boldsymbol{\Sigma}^{-1}(\boldsymbol{X}\boldsymbol{H}_0\boldsymbol{H}_0^\top-\boldsymbol{\Theta})^\top\boldsymbol{R}\\ &\quad+\operatorname{tr}\boldsymbol{\Psi}^2\boldsymbol{R}^\top\boldsymbol{X}\boldsymbol{H}\boldsymbol{H}^\top\boldsymbol{\Sigma}^{-1}\boldsymbol{H}\boldsymbol{H}^\top\boldsymbol{X}^\top\boldsymbol{R}.\end{aligned}$$

Thus the difference in risk of $\widehat{\boldsymbol{\Theta}}_{+}^{SH}$ and $\widehat{\boldsymbol{\Theta}}^{SH}$ is

$$\begin{aligned}&R(\widehat{\boldsymbol{\Theta}}_{+}^{SH},\boldsymbol{\Theta})-R(\widehat{\boldsymbol{\Theta}}^{SH},\boldsymbol{\Theta})\\ &=E[\operatorname{tr}(\boldsymbol{\Psi}_{+}^2-\boldsymbol{\Psi}^2)\boldsymbol{R}^\top\boldsymbol{X}\boldsymbol{H}\boldsymbol{H}^\top\boldsymbol{\Sigma}^{-1}\boldsymbol{H}\boldsymbol{H}^\top\boldsymbol{X}^\top\boldsymbol{R}]\\ &\quad+2E[\operatorname{tr}(\boldsymbol{\Psi}_{+}-\boldsymbol{\Psi})\boldsymbol{R}^\top\boldsymbol{X}\boldsymbol{H}\boldsymbol{H}^\top\boldsymbol{\Sigma}^{-1}(\boldsymbol{X}\boldsymbol{H}_0\boldsymbol{H}_0^\top-\boldsymbol{\Theta})^\top\boldsymbol{R}].\end{aligned}\tag{6.22}$$

The first expectation in the r.h.s. of (6.22) is not positive because $(\psi_i^{+})^2\le\psi_i^2$ for all i.

Recall that $\boldsymbol{S}=\boldsymbol{H}\boldsymbol{L}\boldsymbol{H}^\top$ is the eigenvalue decomposition, where $\boldsymbol{H}\in\mathbb{V}_{p,\nu}$ and $\boldsymbol{L}=\operatorname{diag}(\ell_1,\ldots,\ell_\nu)\in\mathbb{D}_\nu^{(\ge 0)}$. From Proposition 3.2 and Equation (3.3), the joint (unnormalized) p.d.f. of $(\boldsymbol{X},\boldsymbol{L},\boldsymbol{H})$ without a normalizing constant can be written as

$$\exp\Big(-\frac{1}{2}\operatorname{tr}(\boldsymbol{X}-\boldsymbol{\Theta})\boldsymbol{\Sigma}^{-1}(\boldsymbol{X}-\boldsymbol{\Theta})^\top-\frac{1}{2}\operatorname{tr}\boldsymbol{\Sigma}^{-1}\boldsymbol{H}\boldsymbol{L}\boldsymbol{H}^\top\Big)g_{n,p}(\boldsymbol{L}),$$

where

$$g_{n,p}(\boldsymbol{L})=|\boldsymbol{L}|^{(|n-p|-1)/2}\prod_{1\le i<j\le\nu}(\ell_i-\ell_j).$$

Noting that

$$\begin{aligned}\operatorname{tr}(\boldsymbol{X}-\boldsymbol{\Theta})\boldsymbol{\Sigma}^{-1}(\boldsymbol{X}-\boldsymbol{\Theta})^\top &= \operatorname{tr}(\boldsymbol{X}\boldsymbol{H}_0\boldsymbol{H}_0^\top-\boldsymbol{\Theta})\boldsymbol{\Sigma}^{-1}(\boldsymbol{X}\boldsymbol{H}_0\boldsymbol{H}_0^\top-\boldsymbol{\Theta})^\top\\ &\quad+2\operatorname{tr}\boldsymbol{X}\boldsymbol{H}\boldsymbol{H}^\top\boldsymbol{\Sigma}^{-1}(\boldsymbol{X}\boldsymbol{H}_0\boldsymbol{H}_0^\top-\boldsymbol{\Theta})^\top\\ &\quad+\operatorname{tr}\boldsymbol{X}\boldsymbol{H}\boldsymbol{H}^\top\boldsymbol{\Sigma}^{-1}\boldsymbol{H}\boldsymbol{H}^\top\boldsymbol{X}^\top,\end{aligned}$$

we make the transformation $(\boldsymbol{Z},\boldsymbol{Z}_0)=(\boldsymbol{X}\boldsymbol{H}\boldsymbol{L}^{-1/2},\boldsymbol{X}\boldsymbol{H}_0)$. Since, by Lemma 3.2, the Jacobian of the transformation is given by $J[\boldsymbol{X}\to(\boldsymbol{Z},\boldsymbol{Z}_0)]=|\boldsymbol{L}|^{m/2}$, the joint (unnormalized) p.d.f. of $(\boldsymbol{Z},\boldsymbol{Z}_0,\boldsymbol{L},\boldsymbol{H})$ without a normalizing constant is proportional to

$$\begin{aligned}\exp\Big(&-\frac{1}{2}\operatorname{tr}(\boldsymbol{Z}_0\boldsymbol{H}_0^\top-\boldsymbol{\Theta})\boldsymbol{\Sigma}^{-1}(\boldsymbol{Z}_0\boldsymbol{H}_0^\top-\boldsymbol{\Theta})^\top-\operatorname{tr}\boldsymbol{Z}\boldsymbol{L}^{1/2}\boldsymbol{H}^\top\boldsymbol{\Sigma}^{-1}(\boldsymbol{Z}_0\boldsymbol{H}_0^\top-\boldsymbol{\Theta})^\top\\ &-\frac{1}{2}\operatorname{tr}\boldsymbol{Z}\boldsymbol{L}^{1/2}\boldsymbol{H}^\top\boldsymbol{\Sigma}^{-1}\boldsymbol{H}\boldsymbol{L}^{1/2}\boldsymbol{Z}^\top-\frac{1}{2}\operatorname{tr}\boldsymbol{\Sigma}^{-1}\boldsymbol{H}\boldsymbol{L}\boldsymbol{H}^\top\Big)|\boldsymbol{L}|^{m/2}g_{n,p}(\boldsymbol{L}).\end{aligned}$$

Then the second expectation in the r.h.s. of (6.22) becomes

$$K_0 \iiint_{\mathbb{R}^{m\times(p-\nu)}\times\mathbb{D}_\nu^{(\geq 0)}\times\mathbb{V}_{p,\nu}} I \times f(\boldsymbol{Z}_0, \boldsymbol{L}, \boldsymbol{H})|\boldsymbol{L}|^{m/2} g_{n,p}(\boldsymbol{L})(\mathrm{d}\boldsymbol{Z}_0)(\mathrm{d}\boldsymbol{L})(\boldsymbol{H}^\top \mathrm{d}\boldsymbol{H}),$$

where K_0 is a normalizing constant,

$$\begin{aligned} I = &\int_{\mathbb{R}^{m\times\nu}} \mathrm{tr}\,(\boldsymbol{\Psi}_+ - \boldsymbol{\Psi})\boldsymbol{R}^\top \boldsymbol{Z}\boldsymbol{L}^{1/2}\boldsymbol{H}^\top\boldsymbol{\Sigma}^{-1}(\boldsymbol{Z}_0\boldsymbol{H}_0^\top - \boldsymbol{\Theta})^\top \boldsymbol{R} \\ &\times \exp\Big(- \mathrm{tr}\, \boldsymbol{Z}\boldsymbol{L}^{1/2}\boldsymbol{H}^\top\boldsymbol{\Sigma}^{-1}(\boldsymbol{Z}_0\boldsymbol{H}_0^\top - \boldsymbol{\Theta})^\top - \frac{1}{2}\mathrm{tr}\, \boldsymbol{Z}\boldsymbol{L}^{1/2}\boldsymbol{H}^\top\boldsymbol{\Sigma}^{-1}\boldsymbol{H}\boldsymbol{L}^{1/2}\boldsymbol{Z}^\top\Big)(\mathrm{d}\boldsymbol{Z}) \end{aligned}$$

and

$$f(\boldsymbol{Z}_0, \boldsymbol{L}, \boldsymbol{H}) = \exp\Big(- \frac{1}{2}\mathrm{tr}\,(\boldsymbol{Z}_0\boldsymbol{H}_0^\top - \boldsymbol{\Theta})\boldsymbol{\Sigma}^{-1}(\boldsymbol{Z}_0\boldsymbol{H}_0^\top - \boldsymbol{\Theta})^\top - \frac{1}{2}\mathrm{tr}\,\boldsymbol{\Sigma}^{-1}\boldsymbol{H}\boldsymbol{L}\boldsymbol{H}^\top\Big).$$

Hence if it is shown that $I \leq 0$, the proof of Theorem 6.2 will be complete.

We next consider the singular value decomposition $\boldsymbol{Z} = \boldsymbol{R}\boldsymbol{D}\boldsymbol{V}^\top$, where $\boldsymbol{R} \in \mathbb{V}_{m,\tau}$, $\boldsymbol{D} = \mathrm{diag}\,(d_1, \ldots, d_\tau) = \boldsymbol{F}^{1/2} \in \mathbb{D}_\tau^{(\geq 0)}$, $\boldsymbol{V} \in \mathbb{V}_{\nu,\tau}$ and $\tau = m \wedge (n \wedge p) = m \wedge \nu$. From Lemma 3.6, we have

$$\begin{aligned} (\mathrm{d}\boldsymbol{Z}) &= \frac{1}{2^\tau}|\boldsymbol{D}|^{|m-\nu|} \prod_{1\leq i<j\leq\tau} (d_i^2 - d_j^2)(\boldsymbol{R}^\top \mathrm{d}\boldsymbol{R})(\mathrm{d}\boldsymbol{D})(\boldsymbol{V}^\top \mathrm{d}\boldsymbol{V}) \\ &= \frac{1}{2^{2\tau}} g_{m,\nu}(\boldsymbol{F})(\boldsymbol{R}^\top \mathrm{d}\boldsymbol{R})(\mathrm{d}\boldsymbol{F})(\boldsymbol{V}^\top \mathrm{d}\boldsymbol{V}), \end{aligned}$$

where the second equality is verified by the transformation $\boldsymbol{F} = \boldsymbol{D}^2$. Recall that $(\boldsymbol{R}^\top \mathrm{d}\boldsymbol{R})$ and $(\boldsymbol{V}^\top \mathrm{d}\boldsymbol{V})$ are invariant with respect to any orthogonal transformation. For $i = 1, \ldots, \tau$, it is observed that

$$\{\boldsymbol{R}^\top \boldsymbol{Z}\boldsymbol{L}^{1/2}\boldsymbol{H}^\top\boldsymbol{\Sigma}^{-1}(\boldsymbol{Z}_0\boldsymbol{H}_0^\top - \boldsymbol{\Theta})^\top\boldsymbol{R}\}_{ii} = f_i^{1/2}\boldsymbol{v}_i^\top\boldsymbol{L}^{1/2}\boldsymbol{H}^\top\boldsymbol{\Sigma}^{-1}(\boldsymbol{Z}_0\boldsymbol{H}_0^\top - \boldsymbol{\Theta})^\top\boldsymbol{r}_i,$$

where $\boldsymbol{v}_i$ and $\boldsymbol{r}_i$ are the i-th column vectors of $\boldsymbol{V}$ and $\boldsymbol{R}$, respectively. Letting $\boldsymbol{a}_i^\top = f_i^{1/2}\boldsymbol{v}_i^\top\boldsymbol{L}^{1/2}\boldsymbol{H}^\top\boldsymbol{\Sigma}^{-1}(\boldsymbol{Z}_0\boldsymbol{H}_0^\top - \boldsymbol{\Theta})^\top$, we obtain

$$I = \sum_{i=1}^{\tau} \iiint_{\mathbb{V}_{m,\tau}\times\mathbb{D}_\tau^{(\geq 0)}\times\mathbb{V}_{\nu,\tau}} (\psi_i^+ - \psi_i)\boldsymbol{a}_i^\top\boldsymbol{r}_i e^{-\boldsymbol{a}_i^\top\boldsymbol{r}_i} G_i(\boldsymbol{R}^\top \mathrm{d}\boldsymbol{R})(\mathrm{d}\boldsymbol{F})(\boldsymbol{V}^\top \mathrm{d}\boldsymbol{V}), \tag{6.23}$$

where

$$G_i = \exp\Big(- \sum_{j\neq i}^{\tau}\boldsymbol{a}_j^\top\boldsymbol{r}_j - \frac{1}{2}\mathrm{tr}\,\boldsymbol{F}\boldsymbol{V}^\top\boldsymbol{L}^{1/2}\boldsymbol{H}^\top\boldsymbol{\Sigma}^{-1}\boldsymbol{H}\boldsymbol{L}^{1/2}\boldsymbol{V}\Big) \times \frac{1}{2^{2\tau}} g_{m,\nu}(\boldsymbol{F}).$$

For each $i \in \{1, \ldots, \tau\}$, we make the transformation $\boldsymbol{r}_i \to -\boldsymbol{r}_i$. This transformation is equivalent to the orthogonal transformation $\boldsymbol{R} \to \boldsymbol{R}\boldsymbol{O}_i$, where $\boldsymbol{O}_i \in \mathbb{D}_\tau$ such that the i-th diagonal is minus one and the other diagonals are ones. Since $(\boldsymbol{R}^\top \mathrm{d}\boldsymbol{R})$ is invariant with respect to the orthogonal transformation, (6.23) is rewritten as

$$I = \sum_{i=1}^{\tau} \iiint_{\mathbb{V}_{m,\tau}\times\mathbb{D}_\tau^{(\geq 0)}\times\mathbb{V}_{\nu,\tau}} (\psi_i^+ - \psi_i)(-\boldsymbol{a}_i^\top \boldsymbol{r}_i e^{\boldsymbol{a}_i^\top \boldsymbol{r}_i}) G_i (\boldsymbol{R}^\top \mathrm{d}\boldsymbol{R})(\mathrm{d}\boldsymbol{F})(\boldsymbol{V}^\top \mathrm{d}\boldsymbol{V}). \tag{6.24}$$

Adding each side of (6.23) and (6.24) yields

$$2I = \sum_{i=1}^{\tau} \iiint_{\mathbb{V}_{m,\tau}\times\mathbb{D}_\tau^{(\geq 0)}\times\mathbb{V}_{\nu,\tau}} (\psi_i^+ - \psi_i)\boldsymbol{a}_i^\top \boldsymbol{r}_i (e^{-\boldsymbol{a}_i^\top \boldsymbol{r}_i} - e^{\boldsymbol{a}_i^\top \boldsymbol{r}_i}) G_i (\boldsymbol{R}^\top \mathrm{d}\boldsymbol{R})(\mathrm{d}\boldsymbol{F})(\boldsymbol{V}^\top \mathrm{d}\boldsymbol{V}).$$

Since $\psi_i^+ \geq \psi_i$ and $\boldsymbol{a}_i^\top \boldsymbol{r}_i (e^{-\boldsymbol{a}_i^\top \boldsymbol{r}_i} - e^{\boldsymbol{a}_i^\top \boldsymbol{r}_i}) \leq 0$ for any value of $\boldsymbol{a}_i^\top \boldsymbol{r}_i$, it always holds that $I \leq 0$. Thus the proof of Theorem 6.2 is complete. □

For example, the Efron-Morris estimator $\widehat{\boldsymbol{\Theta}}^{EM}$ is dominated by

$$\widehat{\boldsymbol{\Theta}}_+^{EM} = \boldsymbol{X}(\boldsymbol{I}_p - \boldsymbol{S}\boldsymbol{S}^+) + \boldsymbol{R}\boldsymbol{\Psi}_+^{EM}(\boldsymbol{F})\boldsymbol{R}^\top \boldsymbol{X}\boldsymbol{S}\boldsymbol{S}^+,$$

where the i-th diagonal element of $\boldsymbol{\Psi}_+^{EM}(\boldsymbol{F})$ is $\max(0, 1 - c^{EM}/f_i)$. This positive-part rule is extending (6.2) to the unknown covariance case. Also, Theorem 6.2 can be applied to $\widehat{\boldsymbol{\Theta}}^{mEM}$, $\widehat{\boldsymbol{\Theta}}^{ST}$ and $\widehat{\boldsymbol{\Theta}}^{mST}$ given in Sect. 6.5, but the applications are omitted.

6.6.2 Shrinkage Estimation with a Loss Matrix

Next, we look at shrinkage estimation under a loss matrix of the form

$$L_M(\widehat{\boldsymbol{\Theta}}, \boldsymbol{\Theta}|\boldsymbol{\Sigma}) = (\widehat{\boldsymbol{\Theta}} - \boldsymbol{\Theta})\boldsymbol{\Sigma}^{-1}(\widehat{\boldsymbol{\Theta}} - \boldsymbol{\Theta})^\top, \tag{6.25}$$

which is an $m \times m$ symmetric positive semi-definite matrix. The corresponding risk matrix is defined by $R_M(\widehat{\boldsymbol{\Theta}}, \boldsymbol{\Theta}) = E[L_M(\widehat{\boldsymbol{\Theta}}, \boldsymbol{\Theta}|\boldsymbol{\Sigma})]$. The loss matrix (6.25) is used in Bilodeau and Kariya (1989). For a more general loss matrix, see Honda (1991).

Using Theorem 5.1 gives

$$R_M(\widehat{\boldsymbol{\Theta}}^{ML}, \boldsymbol{\Theta}) = E[(\boldsymbol{X} - \boldsymbol{\Theta})\boldsymbol{\Sigma}^{-1}(\boldsymbol{X} - \boldsymbol{\Theta})^\top] = E[\nabla_X(\boldsymbol{X} - \boldsymbol{\Theta})] = p\boldsymbol{I}_m.$$

Thus an estimator $\widehat{\boldsymbol{\Theta}}$ is said to be better than $\widehat{\boldsymbol{\Theta}}^{ML}$ relative to the loss matrix (6.25) if $\widehat{\boldsymbol{\Theta}}$ has a smaller risk matrix than $p\boldsymbol{I}_m$ in the Löwner sense, namely, $R_M(\widehat{\boldsymbol{\Theta}}, \boldsymbol{\Theta}) \preceq p\boldsymbol{I}_m$.

Here, we focus our attention on $\widehat{\boldsymbol{\Theta}}^{SH}$ in (6.11). Denote $\boldsymbol{G} = \boldsymbol{R}\boldsymbol{\Phi}\boldsymbol{R}^\top \boldsymbol{X}$. The risk matrix of $\widehat{\boldsymbol{\Theta}}^{SH}$ is written as

$$\begin{aligned} R_M(\widehat{\boldsymbol{\Theta}}^{SH}, \boldsymbol{\Theta}) = R_M(\widehat{\boldsymbol{\Theta}}^{ML}, \boldsymbol{\Theta}) &- E[(\boldsymbol{X} - \boldsymbol{\Theta})\boldsymbol{\Sigma}^{-1}\boldsymbol{S}\boldsymbol{S}^+\boldsymbol{G}^\top] \\ &- E[\{(\boldsymbol{X} - \boldsymbol{\Theta})\boldsymbol{\Sigma}^{-1}\boldsymbol{S}\boldsymbol{S}^+\boldsymbol{G}^\top\}^\top] + E[\boldsymbol{G}\boldsymbol{S}\boldsymbol{S}^+\boldsymbol{\Sigma}^{-1}\boldsymbol{S}\boldsymbol{S}^+\boldsymbol{G}^\top]. \end{aligned}$$

Using the Stein identity (5.1) gives

$$E[(\boldsymbol{X}-\boldsymbol{\Theta})\boldsymbol{\Sigma}^{-1}\boldsymbol{S}\boldsymbol{S}^{+}\boldsymbol{G}^{\top}] = E[\nabla_X \boldsymbol{S}\boldsymbol{S}^{+}\boldsymbol{G}^{\top}]$$

and

$$\begin{aligned} E[\boldsymbol{G}\boldsymbol{S}\boldsymbol{S}^{+}\boldsymbol{\Sigma}^{-1}\boldsymbol{S}\boldsymbol{S}^{+}\boldsymbol{G}^{\top}] &= E[\boldsymbol{G}\boldsymbol{S}^{+}\boldsymbol{Y}^{\top}\boldsymbol{Y}\boldsymbol{\Sigma}^{-1}\boldsymbol{S}\boldsymbol{S}^{+}\boldsymbol{G}^{\top}] \\ &= E[\boldsymbol{G}\boldsymbol{S}^{+}\boldsymbol{Y}^{\top}\nabla_Y \boldsymbol{S}\boldsymbol{S}^{+}\boldsymbol{G}^{\top}] + E[\{\boldsymbol{G}\boldsymbol{S}\boldsymbol{S}^{+}\nabla_Y^{\top}\boldsymbol{Y}\boldsymbol{S}^{+}\boldsymbol{G}^{\top}\}^{\top}]. \end{aligned}$$

Thus the unbiased risk estimate of $\widehat{\boldsymbol{\Theta}}^{SH}$ relative to the loss matrix (6.25) becomes

$$\begin{aligned} \widehat{R}_M(\widehat{\boldsymbol{\Theta}}^{SH}) = p\boldsymbol{I}_m &- \nabla_X \boldsymbol{S}\boldsymbol{S}^{+}\boldsymbol{G}^{\top} - \{\nabla_X \boldsymbol{S}\boldsymbol{S}^{+}\boldsymbol{G}^{\top}\}^{\top} \\ &+ \boldsymbol{G}\boldsymbol{S}^{+}\boldsymbol{Y}^{\top}\nabla_Y \boldsymbol{S}\boldsymbol{S}^{+}\boldsymbol{G}^{\top} + \{\boldsymbol{G}\boldsymbol{S}\boldsymbol{S}^{+}\nabla_Y^{\top}\boldsymbol{Y}\boldsymbol{S}^{+}\boldsymbol{G}^{\top}\}^{\top}, \end{aligned}$$

implying that, according to Lemmas 6.6 and 6.7 in the Appendix,

$$\widehat{R}_M(\widehat{\boldsymbol{\Theta}}^{SH}) = p\boldsymbol{I}_m - 2(\mathrm{tr}\,\boldsymbol{\Phi})(\boldsymbol{I}_m - \boldsymbol{R}\boldsymbol{R}^{\top}) + \boldsymbol{R}\boldsymbol{\Phi}^{*}\boldsymbol{R}^{\top},$$

where $\boldsymbol{\Phi}^{*} = \mathrm{diag}\,(\phi_1^{*}, \ldots, \phi_\tau^{*})$ and for $i = 1, \ldots, \tau$

$$\begin{aligned} \phi_i^{*} = a f_i \phi_i^2 - 4 f_i^2 \phi_i \frac{\partial \phi_i}{\partial f_i} - 2\sum_{j\neq i}^{\tau} \frac{f_i^2\phi_i^2}{f_i - f_j} + 2\sum_{j\neq i}^{\tau} \frac{f_i\phi_i f_j\phi_j}{f_i - f_j} \\ - 2(n \wedge p - \tau + 1)\phi_i - 4 f_i \frac{\partial \phi_i}{\partial f_i} - 2\sum_{j\neq i}^{\tau} \frac{f_i\phi_i - f_j\phi_j}{f_i - f_j} \end{aligned}$$

with $a = n + p - 2(n \wedge p) + 2\tau - 3 = (|n - p| + 2m) \wedge (n + p) - 3$. The above discussion is summarized as follows.

Proposition 6.1 *If* $\sum_{i=1}^{\tau} \phi_i \geq 0$ *and* $\phi_i^{*} \leq 0$ *for* $i = 1, \ldots, \tau$, *then* $\widehat{\boldsymbol{\Theta}}^{SH}$ *dominates* $\widehat{\boldsymbol{\Theta}}^{ML}$ *relative to the loss matrix* (6.25).

As a specific example, we consider improvement on the Efron-Morris type estimator (6.9). Putting $\phi_i = c/f_i$ gives $\phi_i^{*} = \{(a+4)c^2 - 2(n \wedge p - \tau - 1)\} f_i^{-1}$ for each i. Hence if $\tau = m$ and $0 < c \leq 2(n \wedge p - m - 1)/(a + 4)$, then $\widehat{R}_M(\widehat{\boldsymbol{\Theta}}^{EMK}) \preceq p\boldsymbol{I}_m$.

6.6.3 Application to a GMANOVA Model

Here, we treat shrinkage estimation in a generalized MANOVA model (Potthoff and Roy, 1964) of the form

$$\boldsymbol{Z} = \boldsymbol{A}\boldsymbol{B}\boldsymbol{C} + \boldsymbol{E}, \tag{6.26}$$

where $\boldsymbol{Z} \in \mathbb{R}^{N\times q}$ is an observation matrix, $\boldsymbol{A} \in \mathbb{R}^{N\times m_1}$ and $\boldsymbol{C} \in \mathbb{R}^{p\times q}$ are constant matrices of full rank with $N \geq m_1$ and $q \geq p$, $\boldsymbol{B} \in \mathbb{R}^{m_1\times p}$ is an unknown regression coefficient matrix and $\boldsymbol{E} \in \mathbb{R}^{N\times q}$ is a random error matrix. Assume that $\boldsymbol{E} \sim \mathcal{N}_{N\times q}(\boldsymbol{0}_{N\times q}, \boldsymbol{I}_N \otimes \boldsymbol{\Sigma}_0)$ and $\boldsymbol{\Sigma}_0 \in \mathbb{S}_q^{(+)}$ is unknown. The generalized MANOVA model is abbreviated by the GMANOVA model and it is also called the growth curve model. The purpose of this section is to present a shrinkage estimator of $\boldsymbol{B}$ improving the ML estimator.

To simplify the estimation problem, we first derive a canonical form of (6.26). Let $\boldsymbol{\Gamma}_A \in \mathbb{O}_N$ and $\boldsymbol{\Gamma}_C \in \mathbb{O}_q$ such that

$$\boldsymbol{\Gamma}_A\boldsymbol{A} = \begin{pmatrix} (\boldsymbol{A}^\top\boldsymbol{A})^{1/2} \\ \boldsymbol{0}_{(N-m_1)\times m_1} \end{pmatrix}, \qquad \boldsymbol{C}\boldsymbol{\Gamma}_C = ((\boldsymbol{C}\boldsymbol{C}^\top)^{1/2}, \boldsymbol{0}_{p\times m_2})$$

for $m_2 = q - p$. Denote $\boldsymbol{\Theta} = (\boldsymbol{A}^\top\boldsymbol{A})^{1/2}\boldsymbol{B}(\boldsymbol{C}\boldsymbol{C}^\top)^{1/2}$,

$$\boldsymbol{\Gamma}_A\boldsymbol{Z}\boldsymbol{\Gamma}_C = \begin{pmatrix} \boldsymbol{X}_1 & \boldsymbol{U} \\ \boldsymbol{Z}_1 & \boldsymbol{Z}_2 \end{pmatrix}, \quad \boldsymbol{\Gamma}_C^\top\boldsymbol{\Sigma}_0\boldsymbol{\Gamma}_C = \begin{pmatrix} \boldsymbol{I}_p & \boldsymbol{\Xi}^\top \\ \boldsymbol{0}_{m_2\times p} & \boldsymbol{I}_{m_2} \end{pmatrix} \begin{pmatrix} \boldsymbol{\Sigma} & \boldsymbol{0}_{p\times m_2} \\ \boldsymbol{0}_{m_2\times p} & \boldsymbol{\Omega} \end{pmatrix} \begin{pmatrix} \boldsymbol{I}_p & \boldsymbol{0}_{p\times m_2} \\ \boldsymbol{\Xi} & \boldsymbol{I}_{m_2} \end{pmatrix},$$

where $\boldsymbol{X}_1 \in \mathbb{R}^{m_1\times p}$, $\boldsymbol{U} \in \mathbb{R}^{m_1\times m_2}$, $\boldsymbol{\Sigma} \in \mathbb{S}_p^{(+)}$, $\boldsymbol{\Omega} \in \mathbb{S}_{m_2}^{(+)}$ and $\boldsymbol{\Xi} \in \mathbb{R}^{m_2\times p}$. Further let $\boldsymbol{\Gamma}_Z \in \mathbb{O}_{N-m_1}$ such that

$$\boldsymbol{\Gamma}_Z\boldsymbol{Z}_2 = \begin{pmatrix} \boldsymbol{W}^{1/2} \\ \boldsymbol{0}_{n\times m_2} \end{pmatrix}$$

with $n = N - m_1 - m_2$ and $\boldsymbol{W} = \boldsymbol{Z}_2^\top\boldsymbol{Z}_2$. Denote $\boldsymbol{\Gamma}_Z\boldsymbol{Z}_1 = (\boldsymbol{V}^\top\boldsymbol{W}^{1/2}, \boldsymbol{Y}^\top)^\top$, where $\boldsymbol{V} \in \mathbb{R}^{m_2\times p}$. Then a canonical form of (6.26) is given as follows:

$$\begin{aligned} \boldsymbol{X}_1|\boldsymbol{U} &\sim \mathcal{N}_{m_1\times p}(\boldsymbol{\Theta} + \boldsymbol{U}\boldsymbol{\Xi}, \boldsymbol{I}_{m_1} \otimes \boldsymbol{\Sigma}), && (6.27)\\ \boldsymbol{U} &\sim \mathcal{N}_{m_1\times m_2}(\boldsymbol{0}_{m_1\times m_2}, \boldsymbol{I}_{m_1} \otimes \boldsymbol{\Omega}), && (6.28)\\ \boldsymbol{Y} &\sim \mathcal{N}_{n\times p}(\boldsymbol{0}_{n\times p}, \boldsymbol{I}_n \otimes \boldsymbol{\Sigma}), && (6.29)\\ \boldsymbol{V}|\boldsymbol{W} &\sim \mathcal{N}_{m_2\times p}(\boldsymbol{\Xi}, \boldsymbol{W}^{-1} \otimes \boldsymbol{\Sigma}), && (6.30)\\ \boldsymbol{W} &\sim \mathcal{W}_{m_2}(N - m_1, \boldsymbol{\Omega}), && (6.31) \end{aligned}$$

where $(\boldsymbol{X}_1, \boldsymbol{U})$, $\boldsymbol{Y}$ and $(\boldsymbol{V}, \boldsymbol{W})$ are independent. For derivation of the above canonical form, see Srivastava and Khatri (1979, pp.192–193).

Here we view the estimation problem of $\boldsymbol{\Theta}$ relative to the quadratic loss

$$L(\widehat{\boldsymbol{\Theta}}, \boldsymbol{\Theta}|\boldsymbol{\Sigma}) = \operatorname{tr}(\widehat{\boldsymbol{\Theta}} - \boldsymbol{\Theta})\boldsymbol{\Sigma}^{-1}(\widehat{\boldsymbol{\Theta}} - \boldsymbol{\Theta})^\top. \tag{6.32}$$

The risk is defined by $R(\widehat{\boldsymbol{\Theta}}, \boldsymbol{\Theta}) = E[L(\widehat{\boldsymbol{\Theta}}, \boldsymbol{\Theta}|\boldsymbol{\Sigma})]$, where the expectation is taken with respect to (6.27)–(6.31).

The ML estimator of $\boldsymbol{\Theta}$ is

$$\widehat{\boldsymbol{\Theta}}^{ML} = \boldsymbol{X}_1 - \boldsymbol{U}\boldsymbol{V}.$$

Denote $\boldsymbol{S} = \boldsymbol{Y}^\top \boldsymbol{Y}$. To improve $\widehat{\boldsymbol{\Theta}}^{ML}$, we consider a double shrinkage estimator (Kariya et al. 1996, 1999) having the form

$$\widehat{\boldsymbol{\Theta}}^{DSH} = \boldsymbol{X}_1 - \boldsymbol{G}_1 - \boldsymbol{U}(\boldsymbol{V} - \boldsymbol{G}_2),$$

where $\boldsymbol{G}_1 = \boldsymbol{G}_1(\boldsymbol{X}_1, \boldsymbol{S}) \in \mathbb{R}^{m_1 \times p}$, and $\boldsymbol{G}_2 = \boldsymbol{G}_2(\boldsymbol{V}, \boldsymbol{S}|\boldsymbol{U}, \boldsymbol{W}) \in \mathbb{R}^{m_2 \times p}$ satisfies

$$\boldsymbol{G}_2(\boldsymbol{V}, \boldsymbol{S}|\boldsymbol{U}, \boldsymbol{W}) = \boldsymbol{G}_2(\boldsymbol{V}, \boldsymbol{S}| - \boldsymbol{U}, \boldsymbol{W}). \tag{6.33}$$

The risk of $\widehat{\boldsymbol{\Theta}}^{DSH}$ can be written as

$$\begin{aligned} R(\widehat{\boldsymbol{\Theta}}^{DSH}, \boldsymbol{\Theta}) = {} & E[\operatorname{tr}(\boldsymbol{X}_1 - \boldsymbol{G}_1 - \boldsymbol{\Theta} - \boldsymbol{U}\boldsymbol{\Xi})\boldsymbol{\Sigma}^{-1}(\boldsymbol{X}_1 - \boldsymbol{G}_1 - \boldsymbol{\Theta} - \boldsymbol{U}\boldsymbol{\Xi})] \\ & - 2E[\operatorname{tr}(\boldsymbol{X}_1 - \boldsymbol{G}_1 - \boldsymbol{\Theta} - \boldsymbol{U}\boldsymbol{\Xi})\boldsymbol{\Sigma}^{-1}(\boldsymbol{V} - \boldsymbol{G}_2 - \boldsymbol{\Xi})^\top \boldsymbol{U}^\top] \\ & + E[\operatorname{tr}\boldsymbol{U}(\boldsymbol{V} - \boldsymbol{G}_2 - \boldsymbol{\Xi})\boldsymbol{\Sigma}^{-1}(\boldsymbol{V} - \boldsymbol{G}_2 - \boldsymbol{\Xi})^\top \boldsymbol{U}^\top]. \end{aligned} \tag{6.34}$$

The second term of the r.h.s. in (6.34) is zero because the distributions (6.27), (6.28) and (6.30) are symmetric and $\boldsymbol{G}_2$ has the symmetry assumption (6.33), so that

$$R(\widehat{\boldsymbol{\Theta}}^{DSH}, \boldsymbol{\Theta}) = E^{\boldsymbol{U}}[R_1(\boldsymbol{G}_1)] + E^{\boldsymbol{U},\boldsymbol{W}}[R_2(\boldsymbol{G}_2)],$$

where

$$\begin{aligned} R_1(\boldsymbol{G}_1) &= E[\operatorname{tr}(\boldsymbol{X}_1 - \boldsymbol{G}_1 - \boldsymbol{\Theta} - \boldsymbol{U}\boldsymbol{\Xi})\boldsymbol{\Sigma}^{-1}(\boldsymbol{X}_1 - \boldsymbol{G}_1 - \boldsymbol{\Theta} - \boldsymbol{U}\boldsymbol{\Xi})|\boldsymbol{U}], \\ R_2(\boldsymbol{G}_2) &= E[\operatorname{tr}\boldsymbol{U}^\top \boldsymbol{U}(\boldsymbol{V} - \boldsymbol{G}_2 - \boldsymbol{\Xi})\boldsymbol{\Sigma}^{-1}(\boldsymbol{V} - \boldsymbol{G}_2 - \boldsymbol{\Xi})^\top|\boldsymbol{U}, \boldsymbol{W}]. \end{aligned}$$

This suggests the possibility of double shrinkage estimation in both distributions of $\boldsymbol{X}_1$ and $\boldsymbol{V}$. The risk of the ML estimator can be expressed as $R(\widehat{\boldsymbol{\Theta}}^{ML}, \boldsymbol{\Theta}) = E^{\boldsymbol{U}}[R_1(\boldsymbol{0}_{m_1 \times p})] + E^{\boldsymbol{U},\boldsymbol{W}}[R_2(\boldsymbol{0}_{m_2 \times p})]$.

For example, we consider the case of $m_1 \geq m_2$. Let $\tau_1 = m_1 \wedge n \wedge p$,

$$\boldsymbol{X}_1 \boldsymbol{S}^+ \boldsymbol{X}_1^\top = \boldsymbol{R}_1 \boldsymbol{F}_1 \boldsymbol{R}_1^\top, \quad \boldsymbol{G}_1^{EM} = c_1 \boldsymbol{R}_1 \boldsymbol{F}_1^{-1} \boldsymbol{R}_1^\top \boldsymbol{X}_1 \boldsymbol{S}\boldsymbol{S}^+,$$

where $\boldsymbol{F}_1 \in \mathbb{D}_{\tau_1}^{(\geq 0)}$, $\boldsymbol{R}_1 \in \mathbb{V}_{m_1 \times \tau_1}$ and c_1 is a positive constant. In addition, let $\tau_2 = m_2 \wedge n \wedge p$, $\boldsymbol{X}_2 = (\boldsymbol{U}^\top \boldsymbol{U})^{-1/2} \boldsymbol{W}\boldsymbol{V}$,

$$\boldsymbol{X}_2 \boldsymbol{S}^+ \boldsymbol{X}_2^\top = \boldsymbol{R}_2 \boldsymbol{F}_2 \boldsymbol{R}_2^\top, \quad \boldsymbol{G}_2^{EM} = c_2 (\boldsymbol{U}^\top \boldsymbol{U})^{-1/2} \boldsymbol{R}_2 \boldsymbol{F}_2^{-1} \boldsymbol{R}_2^\top \boldsymbol{X}_2 \boldsymbol{S}\boldsymbol{S}^+,$$

where $\boldsymbol{F}_2 \in \mathbb{D}_{\tau_2}^{(\geq 0)}$, $\boldsymbol{R}_2 \in \mathbb{V}_{m_2 \times \tau_2}$ and c_2 is a positive constant. Then the Efron-Morris type estimator is defined by

$$\widehat{\boldsymbol{\Theta}}^{EM} = \boldsymbol{X}_1 - \boldsymbol{G}_1^{EM} - \boldsymbol{U}(\boldsymbol{V} - \boldsymbol{G}_2^{EM}).$$

Using the same arguments as in Sect. 6.5.1 immediately gives $R_1(\boldsymbol{G}_1^{EM}) \leq R_1(\boldsymbol{0}_{m_1 \times p})$ if

$$0 < c_1 \leq \frac{2(|n \wedge p - m_1| - 1)}{(|n - p| + 2m_1) \wedge (n + p) + 1}. \tag{6.35}$$

For evaluating $R_2(\boldsymbol{G}_2^{EM})$, let ∇_V and ∇_{X_2} be matrix differential operators with respect to $\boldsymbol{V}$ and $\boldsymbol{X}_2$, respectively. Using the same arguments as in (5.2) gives $\nabla_{X_2} = (\boldsymbol{U}^\top \boldsymbol{U})^{1/2} \boldsymbol{W}^{-1} \nabla_V$. The Stein identity (5.1) in terms of (6.30) is used to obtain

$$\begin{aligned}
&E[\operatorname{tr} \boldsymbol{U}^\top \boldsymbol{U}(\boldsymbol{V} - \boldsymbol{\Xi})\boldsymbol{\Sigma}^{-1}(\boldsymbol{G}_2^{EM})^\top | \boldsymbol{U}, \boldsymbol{W}] \\
&= E[\operatorname{tr} \boldsymbol{U}^\top \boldsymbol{U} \boldsymbol{W}^{-1} \nabla_V (\boldsymbol{G}_2^{EM})^\top | \boldsymbol{U}, \boldsymbol{W}] \\
&= c_2 E[\operatorname{tr} (\boldsymbol{U}^\top \boldsymbol{U})^{1/2} \boldsymbol{W}^{-1} \nabla_V \boldsymbol{S}\boldsymbol{S}^+ \boldsymbol{X}_2^\top \boldsymbol{R}_2 \boldsymbol{F}_2^{-1} \boldsymbol{R}_2^\top | \boldsymbol{U}, \boldsymbol{W}] \\
&= c_2 E[\operatorname{tr} \nabla_{X_2} \boldsymbol{S}\boldsymbol{S}^+ \boldsymbol{X}_2^\top \boldsymbol{R}_2 \boldsymbol{F}_2^{-1} \boldsymbol{R}_2^\top | \boldsymbol{U}, \boldsymbol{W}].
\end{aligned}$$

Note also that

$$\begin{aligned}
E[\operatorname{tr} \boldsymbol{U}^\top \boldsymbol{U} \boldsymbol{G}_2^{EM} \boldsymbol{\Sigma}^{-1} (\boldsymbol{G}_2^{EM})^\top | \boldsymbol{U}, \boldsymbol{W}] &= E[\operatorname{tr} \boldsymbol{\Sigma}^{-1} \boldsymbol{S}\boldsymbol{S}^+ \boldsymbol{X}_2^\top \boldsymbol{R}_2 \boldsymbol{F}_2^{-2} \boldsymbol{R}_2^\top \boldsymbol{X}_2 \boldsymbol{S}\boldsymbol{S}^+ | \boldsymbol{U}, \boldsymbol{W}] \\
&= E[\operatorname{tr} \nabla_Y^\top \boldsymbol{Y} \boldsymbol{S}^+ \boldsymbol{X}_2^\top \boldsymbol{R}_2 \boldsymbol{F}_2^{-2} \boldsymbol{R}_2^\top \boldsymbol{X}_2 \boldsymbol{S}\boldsymbol{S}^+ | \boldsymbol{U}, \boldsymbol{W}].
\end{aligned}$$

Hence,

$$\begin{aligned}
R_2(\boldsymbol{G}_2^{EM}) = R_2(\boldsymbol{0}_{m_2 \times p}) &- 2c_2 E[\operatorname{tr} \nabla_{X_2} \boldsymbol{S}\boldsymbol{S}^+ \boldsymbol{X}_2^\top \boldsymbol{R}_2 \boldsymbol{F}_2^{-1} \boldsymbol{R}_2^\top | \boldsymbol{U}, \boldsymbol{W}] \\
&+ c_2^2 E[\operatorname{tr} \nabla_Y^\top \boldsymbol{Y} \boldsymbol{S}^+ \boldsymbol{X}_2^\top \boldsymbol{R}_2 \boldsymbol{F}_2^{-2} \boldsymbol{R}_2^\top \boldsymbol{X}_2 \boldsymbol{S}\boldsymbol{S}^+ | \boldsymbol{U}, \boldsymbol{W}].
\end{aligned}$$

Using the same arguments as in Sects. 6.4 and 6.5.1 gives $R_2(\boldsymbol{G}_2^{EM}) \leq R_2(\boldsymbol{0}_{m_2 \times p})$ if

$$0 < c_2 \leq \frac{2(|n \wedge p - m_2| - 1)}{(|n - p| + 2m_2) \wedge (n + p) + 1}. \tag{6.36}$$

From the abovementioned, $\widehat{\boldsymbol{\Theta}}^{EM}$ dominates $\widehat{\boldsymbol{\Theta}}^{ML}$ relative to the quadratic loss (6.32) if c_1 and c_2 satisfy, respectively, (6.35) and (6.36).

A unified dominance result in the case of $m_2 > m_1$ can be established in a similar way to the case of $m_1 \geq m_2$, but it is omitted. Other approaches to decision-theoretic estimation in the GMANOVA model have been studied by Tan (1991), Kubokawa et al. (1992) and Kariya et al. (1996, 1999).

6.6.4 Generalization in an Elliptically Contoured Model

Consider the multivariate linear model (4.1), but the $N \times p$ random error matrix $\boldsymbol{E}$ is assumed to have a p.d.f. of the form

$$|\boldsymbol{\Sigma}|^{-N/2} g(\operatorname{tr} \boldsymbol{\Sigma}^{-1} \boldsymbol{E}^\top \boldsymbol{E}), \tag{6.37}$$

where g is a nonnegative and nonincreasing function on the nonnegative real line. In general, a probability distribution having the p.d.f. (6.37) is commonly called the elliptically contoured distribution. This section introduces shrinkage estimation in the elliptically contoured distribution model.

Using the orthogonal transformation as in Sect. 4.2, we can rewrite (6.37) as

$$|\boldsymbol{\Sigma}|^{-N/2} g(\operatorname{tr} (\boldsymbol{X} - \boldsymbol{\Theta})\boldsymbol{\Sigma}^{-1}(\boldsymbol{X} - \boldsymbol{\Theta})^\top + \operatorname{tr} \boldsymbol{\Sigma}^{-1} \boldsymbol{Y}^\top \boldsymbol{Y}), \tag{6.38}$$

where $N = m + n$, $\boldsymbol{X} \in \mathbb{R}^{m \times p}$, $\boldsymbol{Y} \in \mathbb{R}^{n \times p}$, $\boldsymbol{\Theta} \in \mathbb{R}^{m \times p}$ and $\boldsymbol{\Sigma} \in \mathbb{S}_p^{(+)}$. Suppose that $\boldsymbol{\Theta}$ and $\boldsymbol{\Sigma}$ are unknown and that, using $\boldsymbol{X}$ and $\boldsymbol{Y}$, we want to decision-theoretically estimate $\boldsymbol{\Theta}$ relative to the quadratic loss (6.7).

Let

$$G(x) = \frac{1}{2} \int_x^\infty g(t) \mathrm{d}t.$$

Denote

$$E^g[u(\boldsymbol{X}, \boldsymbol{Y})] = \iint_{\mathbb{R}^{m \times p} \times \mathbb{R}^{n \times p}} u(\boldsymbol{X}, \boldsymbol{Y}) |\boldsymbol{\Sigma}|^{-N/2} g(w) (\mathrm{d}\boldsymbol{X})(\mathrm{d}\boldsymbol{Y}),$$
$$E^G[u(\boldsymbol{X}, \boldsymbol{Y})] = \iint_{\mathbb{R}^{m \times p} \times \mathbb{R}^{n \times p}} u(\boldsymbol{X}, \boldsymbol{Y}) |\boldsymbol{\Sigma}|^{-N/2} G(w) (\mathrm{d}\boldsymbol{X})(\mathrm{d}\boldsymbol{Y}),$$

where $w = \operatorname{tr} (\boldsymbol{X} - \boldsymbol{\Theta})\boldsymbol{\Sigma}^{-1}(\boldsymbol{X} - \boldsymbol{\Theta})^\top + \operatorname{tr} \boldsymbol{\Sigma}^{-1} \boldsymbol{Y}^\top \boldsymbol{Y}$ and u is an integrable function. Let $\boldsymbol{U} \in \mathbb{R}^{m \times p}$ such that all elements of $\boldsymbol{U}$ are absolutely continuous functions of $\boldsymbol{X}$. Then, under some suitable conditions,

$$E^g[\operatorname{tr} (\boldsymbol{X} - \boldsymbol{\Theta})\boldsymbol{\Sigma}^{-1} \boldsymbol{U}^\top] = E^G[\operatorname{tr} \nabla_X \boldsymbol{U}^\top]. \tag{6.39}$$

For details of the conditions, see Kubokawa and Srivastava (2001). The identity (6.39) is an extension of the Stein identity (5.3).

Applying the Stein identity (6.39) to the risk function of $\widehat{\boldsymbol{\Theta}}^{ML} = \boldsymbol{X}$, we obtain

$$\begin{aligned} R_g(\widehat{\boldsymbol{\Theta}}^{ML}, \boldsymbol{\Theta}) &= E^g[\operatorname{tr} (\boldsymbol{X} - \boldsymbol{\Theta})\boldsymbol{\Sigma}^{-1}(\boldsymbol{X} - \boldsymbol{\Theta})^\top] = E^G[\operatorname{tr} \nabla_X (\boldsymbol{X} - \boldsymbol{\Theta})^\top] \\ &= E^G[mp]. \end{aligned}$$

The risk of $\widehat{\boldsymbol{\Theta}}^{SH}$ in (6.11) is expanded to

$$R_g(\widehat{\boldsymbol{\Theta}}^{SH}, \boldsymbol{\Theta}|\boldsymbol{\Sigma}) = R_g(\widehat{\boldsymbol{\Theta}}^{ML}, \boldsymbol{\Theta}|\boldsymbol{\Sigma}) + E^g[\operatorname{tr} \boldsymbol{R\Phi R}^\top \boldsymbol{XSS}^+\boldsymbol{\Sigma}^{-1}\boldsymbol{SS}^+\boldsymbol{X}^\top \boldsymbol{R\Phi R}^\top - 2\operatorname{tr}(\boldsymbol{X}-\boldsymbol{\Theta})\boldsymbol{\Sigma}^{-1}\boldsymbol{SS}^+\boldsymbol{X}^\top\boldsymbol{R\Phi R}^\top],$$

so that, by the Stein identity (6.39), $R_g(\widehat{\boldsymbol{\Theta}}^{SH}, \boldsymbol{\Theta}|\boldsymbol{\Sigma}) = E^G[\widehat{\Delta}_G^{SH}]$, where

$$\widehat{\Delta}_G^{SH} = mp + \operatorname{tr} \nabla_Y^\top \boldsymbol{YS}^+\boldsymbol{X}^\top\boldsymbol{R\Phi}^2\boldsymbol{R}^\top\boldsymbol{XSS}^+ - 2\operatorname{tr}\nabla_X \boldsymbol{SS}^+\boldsymbol{X}^\top\boldsymbol{R\Phi R}^\top.$$

Although $\widehat{\Delta}_G^{SH}$ is not an unbiased risk estimator for $\widehat{\boldsymbol{\Theta}}^{SH}$, we can see that $\widehat{\boldsymbol{\Theta}}^{SH}$ dominates $\widehat{\boldsymbol{\Theta}}^{ML}$ if $\widehat{\Delta}_G^{SH} \le mp$. Hence the improving procedures in Sect. 6.5 can be applied to estimation of $\boldsymbol{\Theta}$ in (6.38), and the corresponding dominance results hold without depending on the underlying function g.

Appendix

This appendix provides some brief proofs of useful results on matrix differential operators that were previously applied to Theorem 6.1.

Let $\boldsymbol{X} = (x_{ab}) \in \mathbb{R}^{m\times p}$ and $\boldsymbol{Y} = (y_{ab}) \in \mathbb{R}^{n\times p}$. Denote the matrix differential operators with respect to $\boldsymbol{X}$ and $\boldsymbol{Y}$, respectively, by $\nabla_X = (\mathrm{d}_{ab}^X)$ with $\mathrm{d}_{ab}^X = \partial/\partial x_{ab}$ and by $\nabla_Y = (\mathrm{d}_{ab}^Y)$ with $\mathrm{d}_{ab}^Y = \partial/\partial y_{ab}$. Let

$$\tau = m \wedge n \wedge p.$$

Here, the eigenvalue decomposition of $\boldsymbol{XS}^+\boldsymbol{X}^\top$ is

$$\boldsymbol{XS}^+\boldsymbol{X}^\top = \boldsymbol{RFR}^\top,$$

where $\boldsymbol{F} = \operatorname{diag}(f_1, \ldots, f_\tau) \in \mathbb{D}_\tau^{(\ge 0)}$ and $\boldsymbol{R} = (r_{ij}) \in \mathbb{V}_{m,\tau}$.

Lemma 6.5 *For $i = 1, \ldots, \tau$, $k = 1, \ldots, m$, $a = 1, \ldots, m$ and $b = 1, \ldots, p$, we have*

(i) $\mathrm{d}_{ab}^X f_i = A_{ab}^{ii}$,

(ii) $\mathrm{d}_{ab}^X r_{ki} = \sum_{j\neq i}^{\tau} \dfrac{r_{kj}A_{ab}^{ij}}{f_i - f_j} + f_i^{-1}\{\boldsymbol{I}_m - \boldsymbol{RR}^\top\}_{ka}\{\boldsymbol{R}^\top\boldsymbol{XS}^+\}_{ib}$,

where $A_{ab}^{ij} = r_{aj}\{\boldsymbol{R}^\top\boldsymbol{XS}^+\}_{ib} + r_{ai}\{\boldsymbol{R}^\top\boldsymbol{XS}^+\}_{jb}$.

For $i = 1, \ldots, \tau$, $k = 1, \ldots, m$, $a = 1, \ldots, n$ and $b = 1, \ldots, p$, we have

(iii) $\mathrm{d}_{ab}^Y f_i = B_{ab}^{ii}$,

(iv) $\mathrm{d}_{ab}^Y r_{ki} = \sum_{j\neq i}^{\tau} \dfrac{r_{kj}B_{ab}^{ij}}{f_i - f_j} + f_i^{-1}\{\boldsymbol{R}^\top\boldsymbol{XS}^+\boldsymbol{S}^+\boldsymbol{Y}^\top\}_{ia}\{(\boldsymbol{I}_m - \boldsymbol{RR}^\top)\boldsymbol{X}(\boldsymbol{I}_p - \boldsymbol{SS}^+)\}_{kb}$, *where*

$$\begin{aligned}B_{ab}^{ij} &= -\{\boldsymbol{R}^\top\boldsymbol{X}\boldsymbol{S}^+\boldsymbol{Y}^\top\}_{ia}\{\boldsymbol{R}^\top\boldsymbol{X}\boldsymbol{S}^+\}_{jb} - \{\boldsymbol{R}^\top\boldsymbol{X}\boldsymbol{S}^+\boldsymbol{Y}^\top\}_{ja}\{\boldsymbol{R}^\top\boldsymbol{X}\boldsymbol{S}^+\}_{ib}\\ &+ \{\boldsymbol{R}^\top\boldsymbol{X}\boldsymbol{S}^+\boldsymbol{S}^+\boldsymbol{Y}^\top\}_{ia}\{\boldsymbol{R}^\top\boldsymbol{X}(\boldsymbol{I}_p - \boldsymbol{S}\boldsymbol{S}^+)\}_{jb}\\ &+ \{\boldsymbol{R}^\top\boldsymbol{X}\boldsymbol{S}^+\boldsymbol{S}^+\boldsymbol{Y}^\top\}_{ja}\{\boldsymbol{R}^\top\boldsymbol{X}(\boldsymbol{I}_p - \boldsymbol{S}\boldsymbol{S}^+)\}_{ib}.\end{aligned}$$

Proof Take $\boldsymbol{R}_* \in \mathbb{V}_{m,m-\tau}$ such that $\boldsymbol{R}_*^\top\boldsymbol{R} = \boldsymbol{0}_{(m-\tau)\times\tau}$. Define $\boldsymbol{R}_0 = (\boldsymbol{R}, \boldsymbol{R}_*) \in \mathbb{O}_m$. Denote $\boldsymbol{F}_0 = \mathrm{diag}\,(f_1, \dots, f_\tau, 0, \dots, 0)$ $(\in \mathbb{D}_m^{(\geq 0)})$. Then $\boldsymbol{X}\boldsymbol{S}^+\boldsymbol{X}^\top = \boldsymbol{R}_0\boldsymbol{F}_0\boldsymbol{R}_0^\top$.

Differentiating both sides of $\boldsymbol{R}_0^\top\boldsymbol{R}_0 = \boldsymbol{I}_m$ gives $[\mathrm{d}\boldsymbol{R}_0^\top]\boldsymbol{R}_0 + \boldsymbol{R}_0^\top\mathrm{d}\boldsymbol{R}_0 = \boldsymbol{0}_{m\times m}$, implying that $\boldsymbol{R}_0^\top\mathrm{d}\boldsymbol{R}_0$ is skew-symmetric in $\mathbb{R}^{m\times m}$. Thus, for $j, i \in \{1, \dots, m\}$, $\{\boldsymbol{R}_0^\top\mathrm{d}\boldsymbol{R}_0\}_{ji} = 0$ if $j = i$ and $\{\boldsymbol{R}_0^\top\mathrm{d}\boldsymbol{R}_0\}_{ji} = -\{\boldsymbol{R}_0^\top\mathrm{d}\boldsymbol{R}_0\}_{ij} = -\{[\mathrm{d}\boldsymbol{R}_0^\top]\boldsymbol{R}_0\}_{ji}$ otherwise. Differentiating both sides of $\boldsymbol{X}\boldsymbol{S}^+\boldsymbol{X}^\top = \boldsymbol{R}_0\boldsymbol{F}_0\boldsymbol{R}_0^\top$ gives

$$\mathrm{d}(\boldsymbol{X}\boldsymbol{S}^+\boldsymbol{X}^\top) = [\mathrm{d}\boldsymbol{R}_0]\boldsymbol{F}_0\boldsymbol{R}_0^\top + \boldsymbol{R}_0[\mathrm{d}\boldsymbol{F}_0]\boldsymbol{R}_0^\top + \boldsymbol{R}_0\boldsymbol{F}_0\mathrm{d}\boldsymbol{R}_0^\top,$$

and then

$$\begin{aligned}\boldsymbol{R}_0^\top[\mathrm{d}(\boldsymbol{X}\boldsymbol{S}^+\boldsymbol{X}^\top)]\boldsymbol{R}_0 &= [\boldsymbol{R}_0^\top\mathrm{d}\boldsymbol{R}_0]\boldsymbol{F}_0 + \mathrm{d}\boldsymbol{F}_0 + \boldsymbol{F}_0[\mathrm{d}\boldsymbol{R}_0^\top]\boldsymbol{R}_0\\ &= [\boldsymbol{R}_0^\top\mathrm{d}\boldsymbol{R}_0]\boldsymbol{F}_0 + \mathrm{d}\boldsymbol{F}_0 - \boldsymbol{F}_0\boldsymbol{R}_0^\top\mathrm{d}\boldsymbol{R}_0.\end{aligned}$$

Comparing each element in both sides of the above identity, we have

$$\begin{aligned}\mathrm{d}f_i &= \{\boldsymbol{R}^\top[\mathrm{d}(\boldsymbol{X}\boldsymbol{S}^+\boldsymbol{X}^\top)]\boldsymbol{R}\}_{ii} \quad \text{for } i \in \{1, \dots, \tau\},\\ \{\boldsymbol{R}^\top\mathrm{d}\boldsymbol{R}\}_{ji} &= \frac{\{\boldsymbol{R}^\top[\mathrm{d}(\boldsymbol{X}\boldsymbol{S}^+\boldsymbol{X}^\top)]\boldsymbol{R}\}_{ji}}{f_i - f_j} \quad \text{for } j, i \in \{1, \dots, \tau\} \text{ with } j \neq i,\\ \{\boldsymbol{R}_*^\top\mathrm{d}\boldsymbol{R}\}_{ji} &= \frac{\{\boldsymbol{R}_*^\top[\mathrm{d}(\boldsymbol{X}\boldsymbol{S}^+\boldsymbol{X}^\top)]\boldsymbol{R}\}_{ji}}{f_i} \quad \text{for } j \in \{1, \dots, m-\tau\} \text{ and } i \in \{1, \dots, \tau\}.\end{aligned}$$

Note that $\mathrm{d}_{ab}^X\boldsymbol{X} = \boldsymbol{E}_{ab}$, where $\boldsymbol{E}_{ab} \in \mathbb{R}^{m\times p}$ such that the (a, b)-th element is one and the other elements are zeros. Since $\mathrm{d}_{ab}^X(\boldsymbol{X}\boldsymbol{S}^+\boldsymbol{X}^\top) = [\mathrm{d}_{ab}^X\boldsymbol{X}]\boldsymbol{S}^+\boldsymbol{X}^\top + \boldsymbol{X}\boldsymbol{S}^+[\mathrm{d}_{ab}^X\boldsymbol{X}^\top] = \boldsymbol{E}_{ab}\boldsymbol{S}^+\boldsymbol{X}^\top + \boldsymbol{X}\boldsymbol{S}^+\boldsymbol{E}_{ab}^\top$, we observe that, for $j, i \in \{1, \dots, \tau\}$,

$$\begin{aligned}\{\boldsymbol{R}^\top[\mathrm{d}_{ab}^X(\boldsymbol{X}\boldsymbol{S}^+\boldsymbol{X}^\top)]\boldsymbol{R}\}_{ji} &= \{\boldsymbol{R}^\top\boldsymbol{E}_{ab}\boldsymbol{S}^+\boldsymbol{X}^\top\boldsymbol{R}\}_{ji} + \{\boldsymbol{R}^\top\boldsymbol{X}\boldsymbol{S}^+\boldsymbol{E}_{ab}^\top\boldsymbol{R}\}_{ji}\\ &= r_{aj}\{\boldsymbol{S}^+\boldsymbol{X}^\top\boldsymbol{R}\}_{bi} + \{\boldsymbol{R}^\top\boldsymbol{X}\boldsymbol{S}^+\}_{jb}r_{ai} = A_{ab}^{ij}.\end{aligned} \tag{6.40}$$

Thus, for $i = 1, \dots, \tau$, $\mathrm{d}_{ab}^X f_i = \{\boldsymbol{R}^\top[\mathrm{d}_{ab}^X(\boldsymbol{X}\boldsymbol{S}^+\boldsymbol{X}^\top)]\boldsymbol{R}\}_{ii} = A_{ab}^{ii}$, which shows (i).

On the other hand, it is observed that for $k = 1, \dots, m$ and $i = 1, \dots, \tau$

$$
\begin{aligned}
\mathrm{d}^X_{ab} r_{ki} &= \{\mathrm{d}^X_{ab} \boldsymbol{R}\}_{ki} = \{(\boldsymbol{R}\boldsymbol{R}^\top + \boldsymbol{R}_*\boldsymbol{R}_*^\top)\mathrm{d}^X_{ab}\boldsymbol{R}\}_{ki} \\
&= \sum_{j \neq i}^{\tau} r_{kj}\{\boldsymbol{R}^\top \mathrm{d}^X_{ab}\boldsymbol{R}\}_{ji} + \{\boldsymbol{R}_*\boldsymbol{R}_*^\top \mathrm{d}^X_{ab}\boldsymbol{R}\}_{ki} \\
&= \sum_{j \neq i}^{\tau} \frac{r_{kj} A^{ij}_{ab}}{f_i - f_j} + \frac{\{\boldsymbol{R}_*\boldsymbol{R}_*^\top[\mathrm{d}^X_{ab}(\boldsymbol{X}\boldsymbol{S}^+\boldsymbol{X}^\top)]\boldsymbol{R}\}_{ki}}{f_i}.
\end{aligned} \tag{6.41}
$$

In a similar way to (6.40), for $k = 1, \ldots, m$ and $i = 1, \ldots, \tau$,

$$
\{\boldsymbol{R}_*\boldsymbol{R}_*^\top[\mathrm{d}^X_{ab}(\boldsymbol{X}\boldsymbol{S}^+\boldsymbol{X}^\top)]\boldsymbol{R}\}_{ki} = \{\boldsymbol{R}_*\boldsymbol{R}_*^\top\}_{ka}\{\boldsymbol{S}^+\boldsymbol{X}^\top\boldsymbol{R}\}_{bi} + \{\boldsymbol{R}_*\boldsymbol{R}_*^\top\boldsymbol{X}\boldsymbol{S}^+\}_{kb} r_{ai}.
$$

Here, $\boldsymbol{R}_*^\top\boldsymbol{X}\boldsymbol{S}^+ = \boldsymbol{0}_{(m-\tau)\times p}$, so that

$$
\{\boldsymbol{R}_*\boldsymbol{R}_*^\top[\mathrm{d}^X_{ab}(\boldsymbol{X}\boldsymbol{S}^+\boldsymbol{X}^\top)]\boldsymbol{R}\}_{ki} = \{\boldsymbol{I}_m - \boldsymbol{R}\boldsymbol{R}^\top\}_{ka}\{\boldsymbol{R}^\top\boldsymbol{X}\boldsymbol{S}^+\}_{ib}. \tag{6.42}
$$

Substituting (6.42) into (6.41), we obtain (ii).

Since $\{\boldsymbol{R}^\top[\mathrm{d}^Y_{ab}(\boldsymbol{X}\boldsymbol{S}^+\boldsymbol{X}^\top)]\boldsymbol{R}\}_{ji} = \{\boldsymbol{R}^\top\boldsymbol{X}[\mathrm{d}^Y_{ab}\boldsymbol{S}^+]\boldsymbol{X}^\top\boldsymbol{R}\}_{ji}$ for $j, i \in \{1, \ldots, \tau\}$, it is observed from (iii) of Lemma 5.2 that

$$
\begin{aligned}
&\{\boldsymbol{R}^\top[\mathrm{d}^Y_{ab}(\boldsymbol{X}\boldsymbol{S}^+\boldsymbol{X}^\top)]\boldsymbol{R}\}_{ji} \\
&= -\{\boldsymbol{R}^\top\boldsymbol{X}\boldsymbol{S}^+\}_{jb}\{\boldsymbol{R}^\top\boldsymbol{X}\boldsymbol{S}^+\boldsymbol{Y}^\top\}_{ia} - \{\boldsymbol{R}^\top\boldsymbol{X}\boldsymbol{S}^+\boldsymbol{Y}^\top\}_{ja}\{\boldsymbol{R}^\top\boldsymbol{X}\boldsymbol{S}^+\}_{ib} \\
&\quad + \{\boldsymbol{R}^\top\boldsymbol{X}(\boldsymbol{I}_p - \boldsymbol{S}\boldsymbol{S}^+)\}_{jb}\{\boldsymbol{R}^\top\boldsymbol{X}\boldsymbol{S}^+\boldsymbol{S}^+\boldsymbol{Y}^\top\}_{ia} \\
&\quad + \{\boldsymbol{R}^\top\boldsymbol{X}\boldsymbol{S}^+\boldsymbol{S}^+\boldsymbol{Y}^\top\}_{ja}\{\boldsymbol{R}^\top\boldsymbol{X}(\boldsymbol{I}_p - \boldsymbol{S}\boldsymbol{S}^+)\}_{ib} = B^{ij}_{ab}.
\end{aligned}
$$

Similarly,

$$
\{\boldsymbol{R}_*\boldsymbol{R}_*^\top[\mathrm{d}^Y_{ab}(\boldsymbol{X}\boldsymbol{S}^+\boldsymbol{X}^\top)]\boldsymbol{R}\}_{ki} = \{\boldsymbol{R}^\top\boldsymbol{X}\boldsymbol{S}^+\boldsymbol{S}^+\boldsymbol{Y}^\top\}_{ia}\{(\boldsymbol{I}_m - \boldsymbol{R}\boldsymbol{R}^\top)\boldsymbol{X}(\boldsymbol{I}_p - \boldsymbol{S}\boldsymbol{S}^+)\}_{kb}
$$

for $k = 1, \ldots, m$ and $i = 1, \ldots, \tau$. Hence using the same arguments as in the proofs of (i) and (ii) yields (iii) and (iv). □

Lemma 6.6 *Let $c_0 = |n \wedge p - m| + 1$. Define $\boldsymbol{\Phi} = \mathrm{diag}\,(\phi_1, \ldots, \phi_\tau) \in \mathbb{D}_\tau$ such that the diagonals of $\boldsymbol{\Phi}$ are absolutely continuous functions of $\boldsymbol{F}$. Then*

$$
\nabla_X \boldsymbol{S}\boldsymbol{S}^+\boldsymbol{X}^\top\boldsymbol{R}\boldsymbol{\Phi}\boldsymbol{R}^\top = \boldsymbol{R}\boldsymbol{\Phi}^*\boldsymbol{R}^\top + (\mathrm{tr}\,\boldsymbol{\Phi})(\boldsymbol{I}_m - \boldsymbol{R}\boldsymbol{R}^\top), \tag{6.43}
$$

where $\boldsymbol{\Phi}^* = \mathrm{diag}\,(\phi_1^*, \ldots, \phi_\tau^*)$ and for $i = 1, \ldots, \tau$

$$
\phi_i^* = (n \wedge p - \tau + 1)\phi_i + 2f_i\frac{\partial \phi_i}{\partial f_i} + \sum_{j \neq i}^{\tau} \frac{f_i\phi_i - f_j\phi_j}{f_i - f_j}.
$$

In particular,

$$\mathrm{tr}\,\nabla_X \boldsymbol{S}\boldsymbol{S}^+\boldsymbol{X}^\top \boldsymbol{R}\boldsymbol{\Phi}\boldsymbol{R}^\top = \sum_{i=1}^{\tau}\left\{c_0\phi_i + 2f_i\frac{\partial \phi_i}{\partial f_i} + 2\sum_{j>i}^{\tau}\frac{f_i\phi_i - f_j\phi_j}{f_i - f_j}\right\}. \tag{6.44}$$

Proof For $a, c \in \{1, \dots, \tau\}$, the (a, c)-th element of $\nabla_X \boldsymbol{S}\boldsymbol{S}^+\boldsymbol{X}^\top \boldsymbol{R}\boldsymbol{\Phi}\boldsymbol{R}^\top$ is

$$\{\nabla_X \boldsymbol{S}\boldsymbol{S}^+\boldsymbol{X}^\top \boldsymbol{R}\boldsymbol{\Phi}\boldsymbol{R}^\top\}_{ac} = \sum_{b=1}^{p}\sum_{d=1}^{p}\sum_{k=1}^{m}\sum_{i=1}^{\tau} \mathrm{d}_{ab}^X[\{\boldsymbol{S}\boldsymbol{S}^+\}_{bd}x_{kd}r_{ki}\phi_i r_{ci}],$$

and then

$$\{\nabla_X \boldsymbol{S}\boldsymbol{S}^+\boldsymbol{X}^\top \boldsymbol{R}\boldsymbol{\Phi}\boldsymbol{R}^\top\}_{ac} = D_{ac}^{(1)} + D_{ac}^{(2)} + D_{bc}^{(3)}, \tag{6.45}$$

where

$$D_{ac}^{(1)} = \sum_{b=1}^{p}\sum_{d=1}^{p}\sum_{k=1}^{m}\{\boldsymbol{S}\boldsymbol{S}^+\}_{bd}\{\boldsymbol{R}\boldsymbol{\Phi}\boldsymbol{R}^\top\}_{kc}\mathrm{d}_{ab}^X x_{kd},$$

$$D_{ac}^{(2)} = \sum_{b=1}^{p}\sum_{i=1}^{\tau}\{\boldsymbol{S}\boldsymbol{S}^+\boldsymbol{X}^\top \boldsymbol{R}\}_{bi}r_{ci}\mathrm{d}_{ab}^X\phi_i,$$

$$D_{ac}^{(3)} = \sum_{b=1}^{p}\sum_{k=1}^{m}\sum_{i=1}^{\tau}\{\boldsymbol{S}\boldsymbol{S}^+\boldsymbol{X}^\top\}_{bk}\phi_i(r_{ci}\mathrm{d}_{ab}^X r_{ki} + r_{ki}\mathrm{d}_{ab}^X r_{ci}).$$

Since $\mathrm{d}_{ab}^X x_{kd} = \delta_{ak}\delta_{bd}$ and $\boldsymbol{S}\boldsymbol{S}^+$ is idempotent with rank $n \wedge p$, it follows that

$$D_{ac}^{(1)} = \sum_{b=1}^{p}\{\boldsymbol{S}\boldsymbol{S}^+\}_{bb}\{\boldsymbol{R}\boldsymbol{\Phi}\boldsymbol{R}^\top\}_{ac} = (n \wedge p)\{\boldsymbol{R}\boldsymbol{\Phi}\boldsymbol{R}^\top\}_{ac}. \tag{6.46}$$

To evaluate $D_{ac}^{(2)}$, we first use the chain rule and (i) of Lemma 6.5 to obtain

$$\mathrm{d}_{ab}^X\phi_i = \sum_{j=1}^{\tau}[\mathrm{d}_{ab}^X f_j]\frac{\partial \phi_i}{\partial f_j} = \sum_{j=1}^{\tau}A_{ab}^{jj}\frac{\partial \phi_i}{\partial f_j}.$$

Note that $\boldsymbol{S}^+\boldsymbol{S}\boldsymbol{S}^+ = \boldsymbol{S}^+$ and

$$\sum_{b=1}^{p}\{\boldsymbol{S}\boldsymbol{S}^+\boldsymbol{X}^\top \boldsymbol{R}\}_{bi}A_{ab}^{jj} = 2r_{aj}\{\boldsymbol{R}^\top\boldsymbol{X}\boldsymbol{S}^+\boldsymbol{X}^\top\boldsymbol{R}\}_{ji} = 2r_{aj}\{\boldsymbol{F}\}_{ji},$$

so that

$$D_{ac}^{(2)} = 2\sum_{i=1}^{\tau}\sum_{j=1}^{\tau} r_{aj}r_{ci}\{\boldsymbol{F}\}_{ji}\frac{\partial \phi_i}{\partial f_j} = 2\sum_{i=1}^{\tau} r_{ai}r_{ci} f_i \frac{\partial \phi_i}{\partial f_i}. \tag{6.47}$$

Finally, we consider $D_{ac}^{(3)}$. Using (ii) of Lemma 6.5 yields

$$\sum_{k=1}^{m}\{\boldsymbol{S}\boldsymbol{S}^{+}\boldsymbol{X}^{\top}\}_{bk}\mathrm{d}_{ab}^{X} r_{ki} = \sum_{j\neq i}^{\tau}\frac{\{\boldsymbol{S}\boldsymbol{S}^{+}\boldsymbol{X}^{\top}\boldsymbol{R}\}_{bj}A_{ab}^{ij}}{f_i - f_j} + f_i^{-1}\{(\boldsymbol{I}_m - \boldsymbol{R}\boldsymbol{R}^{\top})\boldsymbol{X}\boldsymbol{S}\boldsymbol{S}^{+}\}_{ab}\{\boldsymbol{R}^{\top}\boldsymbol{X}\boldsymbol{S}^{+}\}_{ib}.$$

Since

$$\sum_{b=1}^{p}\{\boldsymbol{S}\boldsymbol{S}^{+}\boldsymbol{X}^{\top}\boldsymbol{R}\}_{bj}A_{ab}^{ij} = r_{aj}\{\boldsymbol{F}\}_{ij} + r_{ai}f_j,$$

$$\sum_{b=1}^{p}\{(\boldsymbol{I}_m - \boldsymbol{R}\boldsymbol{R}^{\top})\boldsymbol{X}\boldsymbol{S}\boldsymbol{S}^{+}\}_{ab}\{\boldsymbol{R}^{\top}\boldsymbol{X}\boldsymbol{S}^{+}\}_{ib} = \{(\boldsymbol{I}_m - \boldsymbol{R}\boldsymbol{R}^{\top})\boldsymbol{X}\boldsymbol{S}^{+}\boldsymbol{X}^{\top}\boldsymbol{R}\}_{ai} = 0,$$

it is seen that

$$\begin{aligned}
&\sum_{b=1}^{p}\sum_{k=1}^{m}\sum_{i=1}^{\tau}\{\boldsymbol{S}\boldsymbol{S}^{+}\boldsymbol{X}^{\top}\}_{bk}\phi_i r_{ci}\mathrm{d}_{ab}^{X} r_{ki}\\
&= \sum_{i=1}^{\tau}\sum_{j\neq i}^{\tau}\frac{r_{ai}r_{ci}f_j\phi_i}{f_i - f_j} = \sum_{i=1}^{\tau}\sum_{j\neq i}^{\tau}\frac{r_{ai}r_{ci}(f_j - f_i + f_i)\phi_i}{f_i - f_j}\\
&= -(\tau-1)\sum_{i=1}^{\tau} r_{ai}r_{ci}\phi_i + \sum_{i=1}^{\tau}\sum_{j\neq i}^{\tau}\frac{r_{ai}r_{ci}f_i\phi_i}{f_i - f_j}.
\end{aligned} \tag{6.48}$$

Similarly,

$$\begin{aligned}
\sum_{b=1}^{p}\sum_{k=1}^{m}\sum_{i=1}^{\tau}\{\boldsymbol{S}\boldsymbol{S}^{+}\boldsymbol{X}^{\top}\}_{bk}\phi_i r_{ki}\mathrm{d}_{ab}^{X} r_{ci} &= \sum_{i=1}^{\tau}\sum_{j\neq i}^{\tau}\frac{r_{aj}r_{cj}f_i\phi_i}{f_i - f_j} + (\mathrm{tr}\,\boldsymbol{\Phi})\{\boldsymbol{I}_m - \boldsymbol{R}\boldsymbol{R}^{\top}\}_{ac}\\
&= -\sum_{i=1}^{\tau}\sum_{j\neq i}^{\tau}\frac{r_{ai}r_{ci}f_j\phi_j}{f_i - f_j} + (\mathrm{tr}\,\boldsymbol{\Phi})\{\boldsymbol{I}_m - \boldsymbol{R}\boldsymbol{R}^{\top}\}_{ac}.
\end{aligned} \tag{6.49}$$

Combining (6.48) and (6.49) gives

$$D_{ac}^{(3)} = \sum_{i=1}^{\tau} r_{ai} r_{ci} \left\{ -(\tau-1)\phi_i + \sum_{j \neq i}^{\tau} \frac{f_i\phi_i - f_j\phi_j}{f_i - f_j} \right\} + (\operatorname{tr} \boldsymbol{\Phi})\{\boldsymbol{I}_m - \boldsymbol{R}\boldsymbol{R}^\top\}_{ac}. \tag{6.50}$$

Substituting (6.46), (6.47) and (6.50) into (6.45) yields (6.43).

Note that $n \wedge p - \tau + 1 + \operatorname{tr}(\boldsymbol{I}_m - \boldsymbol{R}\boldsymbol{R}^\top) = n \wedge p + m - 2\tau + 1 = |n \wedge p - m| + 1 = c_0$ and also that

$$\sum_{i=1}^{\tau} \sum_{j \neq i}^{\tau} \frac{f_i\phi_i - f_j\phi_j}{f_i - f_j} = 2 \sum_{i=1}^{\tau} \sum_{j > i}^{\tau} \frac{f_i\phi_i - f_j\phi_j}{f_i - f_j}.$$

Hence taking the trace of (6.43) yields (6.44), which completes the proof. □

Lemma 6.7 *Let* $c_1 = n - (n \wedge p) + \tau - 2$, $c_2 = p - (n \wedge p) + \tau - 1$ *and* $c_0 = c_1 + c_2$. *Let* $\boldsymbol{\Phi} = \boldsymbol{\Phi}(\boldsymbol{F}) = \operatorname{diag}(\phi_1, \ldots, \phi_\tau)$, *where the* ϕ_i*'s are absolutely continuous functions of* $\boldsymbol{F}$. *Then*

$$\boldsymbol{R}\boldsymbol{\Phi}\boldsymbol{R}^\top \boldsymbol{X}\boldsymbol{S}\boldsymbol{S}^+ \nabla_Y^\top \boldsymbol{Y}\boldsymbol{S}^+ \boldsymbol{X}^\top \boldsymbol{R}\boldsymbol{\Phi}\boldsymbol{R}^\top = \boldsymbol{R}\boldsymbol{\Phi}^{*1}\boldsymbol{R}^\top, \tag{6.51}$$

$$\boldsymbol{R}\boldsymbol{\Phi}\boldsymbol{R}^\top \boldsymbol{X}\boldsymbol{S}^+ \boldsymbol{Y}^\top \nabla_Y \boldsymbol{S}\boldsymbol{S}^+ \boldsymbol{X}^\top \boldsymbol{R}\boldsymbol{\Phi}\boldsymbol{R}^\top = \boldsymbol{R}\boldsymbol{\Phi}^{*2}\boldsymbol{R}^\top, \tag{6.52}$$

where $\boldsymbol{\Phi}^{*k} = \operatorname{diag}(\phi_1^{*k}, \ldots, \phi_\tau^{*k})$ *for* $k = 1, 2$ *and, for* $i = 1, \ldots, \tau$,

$$\phi_i^{*k} = c_k f_i \phi_i^2 - 2 f_i^2 \phi_i \frac{\partial \phi_i}{\partial f_i} - \sum_{j \neq i}^{\tau} \frac{f_i^2 \phi_i^2}{f_i - f_j} + \sum_{j \neq i}^{\tau} \frac{f_i \phi_i f_j \phi_j}{f_i - f_j}.$$

In particular,

$$\operatorname{tr} \nabla_Y^\top \boldsymbol{Y}\boldsymbol{S}^+ \boldsymbol{X}^\top \boldsymbol{R}\boldsymbol{\Phi}^2 \boldsymbol{R}^\top \boldsymbol{X}\boldsymbol{S}\boldsymbol{S}^+ = \sum_{i=1}^{\tau} \left\{ c_0 f_i \phi_i^2 - 2 f_i^2 \frac{\partial(\phi_i^2)}{\partial f_i} - 2 \sum_{j > i}^{\tau} \frac{f_i^2\phi_i^2 - f_j^2\phi_j^2}{f_i - f_j} \right\}. \tag{6.53}$$

Proof The proofs of (6.51) and (6.52) can be done by using the same arguments as in the proof of Lemma 6.6. Since

$$\begin{aligned}
\operatorname{tr} \nabla_Y^\top \boldsymbol{Y}\boldsymbol{S}^+ \boldsymbol{X}^\top \boldsymbol{R}\boldsymbol{\Phi}^2 \boldsymbol{R}^\top \boldsymbol{X}\boldsymbol{S}\boldsymbol{S}^+ &= \operatorname{tr} \nabla_Y^\top \{\boldsymbol{Y}\boldsymbol{S}^+ \boldsymbol{X}^\top \boldsymbol{R}\boldsymbol{\Phi}\boldsymbol{R}^\top \cdot \boldsymbol{R}\boldsymbol{\Phi}\boldsymbol{R}^\top \boldsymbol{X}\boldsymbol{S}\boldsymbol{S}^+\} \\
&= \operatorname{tr} \boldsymbol{R}\boldsymbol{\Phi}\boldsymbol{R}^\top \boldsymbol{X}\boldsymbol{S}\boldsymbol{S}^+ \nabla_Y^\top \boldsymbol{Y}\boldsymbol{S}^+ \boldsymbol{X}^\top \boldsymbol{R}\boldsymbol{\Phi}\boldsymbol{R}^\top \\
&\quad + \operatorname{tr} \boldsymbol{R}\boldsymbol{\Phi}\boldsymbol{R}^\top \boldsymbol{X}\boldsymbol{S}^+ \boldsymbol{Y}^\top \nabla_Y \boldsymbol{S}\boldsymbol{S}^+ \boldsymbol{X}^\top \boldsymbol{R}\boldsymbol{\Phi}\boldsymbol{R}^\top,
\end{aligned}$$

the identity (6.53) can be verified by combining (6.51) and (6.52). □

References

A.J. Baranchik, A family of minimax estimators of the mean of a multivariate normal distribution. Ann. Math. Stat. **41**, 642–645 (1970)

M. Bilodeau, T. Kariya, Minimax estimators in the normal MANOVA model. J. Multivar. Anal. **28**, 260–270 (1989)

D. Chételat, M.T. Wells, Improved multivariate normal mean estimation with unknown covariance when p is greater than n. Ann. Stat. **40**, 3137–3160 (2012)

B. Efron, C. Morris, Empirical Bayes on vector observations: an extension of Stein's method. Biometrika **59**, 335–347 (1972)

B. Efron, C. Morris, Multivariate empirical Bayes and estimation of covariance matrices. Ann. Stat. **4**, 22–32 (1976)

M.H.J. Gruber, *Improving Efficiency by Shrinkage* (Marcel Dekker, New York, 1998)

T. Honda, Minimax estimators in the manova model for arbitrary quadratic loss and unknown covariance matrix. J. Multivar. Anal. **36**, 113–120 (1991)

James, W. and Stein, C. (1961). Estimation with quadratic loss, in *Proceedings of the Fourth Berkeley Symposium on Mathematical Statistics and Probability*, vol. 1, ed. by J. Neyman (University of California Press, Berkeley), pp. 361–379

T. Kariya, Y. Konno, W.E. Strawderman, Double shrinkage estimators in the GMANOVA model. J. Multivar. Anal. **56**, 245–258 (1996)

T. Kariya, Y. Konno, W.E. Strawderman, Construction of shrinkage estimators for the regression coefficient matrix in the GMANOVA model. Commun. Stat.—Theory Methods **28**, 597–611 (1999)

Y. Konno, Families of minimax estimators of matrix of normal means with unknown covariance matrix. J. Japan Stat. Soc. **20**, 191–201 (1990)

Y. Konno, On estimation of a matrix of normal means with unknown covariance matrix. J. Multivar. Anal. **36**, 44–55 (1991)

Y. Konno, Improved estimation of matrix of normal mean and eigenvalues in the multivariate F-distribution. Doctoral dissertation, Institute of Mathematics, University of Tsukuba, 1992. (http://mcm-www.jwu.ac.jp/~konno/)

T. Kubokawa, AKMdE Saleh, K. Morita, Improving on MLE of coefficient matrix in a growth curve model. J. Stat. Plann. Infer. **31**, 169–177 (1992)

T. Kubokawa, M.S. Srivastava, Robust improvement in estimation of a mean matrix in an elliptically contoured distribution. J. Multivar. Anal. **76**, 138–152 (2001)

R.F. Potthoff, S.N. Roy, A generalized multivariate analysis of variance model useful especially for growth curve problems. Biometrika **51**, 313–326 (1964)

M.S. Srivastava, C.G. Khatri, *An Introduction to Multivariate Statistics* (North Holland, New York, 1979)

C. Stein, Estimation of the mean of a multivariate normal distribution. Technical Reports No. 48 (Department of Statistics, Stanford University, Stanford, 1973)

M. Tan, Improved estimators for the GMANOVA problem with application to Monte Carlo simulation. J. Multivar. Anal. **38**, 262–274 (1991)

H. Tsukuma, Shrinkage minimax estimation and positive-part rule for a mean matrix in an elliptically contoured distribution. Stat. Probab. Lett. **80**, 215–220 (2010)

H. Tsukuma, T. Kubokawa, Methods for improvement in estimation of a normal mean matrix. J. Multivar. Anal. **98**, 1592–1610 (2007)

H. Tsukuma, T. Kubokawa, A unified approach to estimating a normal mean matrix in high and low dimensions. J. Multivar. Anal. **139**, 312–328 (2015)

Chapter 7
Estimation of the Covariance Matrix

This chapter addresses decision-theoretic estimation of an error covariance matrix in a multivariate linear model relative to a Stein-type entropy loss. With a unified treatment for high- and low-dimensions, some important improving methods of the best scale and the best triangular invariant estimators are discussed by using the residual sum of squares matrix only. Also this chapter provides interesting dominance results by using the information on both the residual sum of squares matrix and the least squares estimator of the regression coefficient matrix.

7.1 Introduction

As seen in (4.2), a canonical form of multivariate linear model (4.1) is given by

$$\boldsymbol{Y} \sim \mathcal{N}_{n\times p}(\boldsymbol{0}_{n\times p}, \boldsymbol{I}_n \otimes \boldsymbol{\Sigma}), \qquad \boldsymbol{X} \sim \mathcal{N}_{m\times p}(\boldsymbol{\Theta}, \boldsymbol{I}_m \otimes \boldsymbol{\Sigma}),$$

where $\boldsymbol{Y}$ and $\boldsymbol{X}$ are mutually independent, and $\boldsymbol{\Theta} \in \mathbb{R}^{m\times p}$ and $\boldsymbol{\Sigma} \in \mathbb{S}_p^{(+)}$ are matrices of unknown parameters. Throughout this chapter, we use the following notation:

$$\nu = n \wedge p, \qquad \kappa = n \vee p.$$

Here the Wishart matrix $\boldsymbol{S} = \boldsymbol{Y}^\top \boldsymbol{Y}$ is of rank ν and the above canonical form is replaced by

$$\boldsymbol{S} \sim \mathcal{W}_p^{\nu}(n, \boldsymbol{\Sigma}), \qquad \boldsymbol{X} \sim \mathcal{N}_{m\times p}(\boldsymbol{\Theta}, \boldsymbol{I}_m \otimes \boldsymbol{\Sigma}). \tag{7.1}$$

The problem of estimating the covariance matrix $\boldsymbol{\Sigma}$ in (7.1) is looked at from a decision-theoretic point of view.

H. Tsukuma and T. Kubokawa, *Shrinkage Estimation for Mean and Covariance Matrices*, JSS Research Series in Statistics, https://doi.org/10.1007/978-981-15-1596-5_7

In the literature, several loss functions have been employed for decision-theoretic estimation of $\boldsymbol{\Sigma}$ with $n \geq p$. One of such loss functions is Stein's (1956) entropy loss

$$L_S(\widehat{\boldsymbol{\Sigma}}, \boldsymbol{\Sigma}) = \operatorname{tr} \boldsymbol{\Sigma}^{-1}\widehat{\boldsymbol{\Sigma}} - \log |\boldsymbol{\Sigma}^{-1}\widehat{\boldsymbol{\Sigma}}| - p. \tag{7.2}$$

Stein (1956) focused on triangular invariant estimators and succeeded in deriving a minimax estimator improving the sample covariance matrix relative to the loss (7.2). Note that Stein's (1956) results were summarized in James and Stein (1961) and, in this chapter, the minimax estimator is called James and Stein's minimax estimator. Although James and Stein's minimax estimator dominates the sample covariance matrix, the minimax estimator depends on the coordinate system and the dependence causes inadmissibility of the minimax estimator. Typical improved estimators on James and Stein's minimax estimator are orthogonally invariant estimators, which are not influenced by the coordinate system. The orthogonally invariant estimators have been studied since Stein (1975, 1977). For other studies on orthogonally invariant estimators, see Takemura (1984), Dey and Srinivasan (1985), Sheena and Takemura (1992) and Perron (1992).

James and Stein's minimax estimator and its improved estimators mentioned above are based only on $\boldsymbol{S} = \boldsymbol{Y}^\top \boldsymbol{Y}$, while truncation rules have been proposed for improving the existing estimators by using the information contained in $\boldsymbol{X}$. Such a truncation rule was first derived by Stein (1964) in estimation of variance of a normal distribution, and several extensions to multivariate models were studied by Sinha and Ghosh (1987), Perron (1990), Kubokawa et al. (1992) and Kubokawa and Srivastava (2003) in the $n \geq p$ case. These articles applied conditional arguments to deriving dominance results, but Kubokawa and Tsai (2006) used the Stein identity (5.3) to suggest an alternative truncation rule with shrinkage.

When $p > n$, Konno (2009) studied decision-theoretic covariance estimation relative to a quadratic loss. In the $p > n$ case, the Stein loss (7.2) is not available for singular estimators such as the unbiased estimator $\boldsymbol{S}/n$ since $|\boldsymbol{\Sigma}^{-1}\boldsymbol{S}| = 0$. An extended Stein-type entropy loss applicable to singular estimators was treated by Tsukuma (2016a) and Tsukuma and Kubokawa (2016).

This chapter will take a unified approach to both cases of $n \geq p$ and $p > n$. We assume that any estimator lies in $\mathbb{S}_{p,\nu}^{(+)}$ and it is of the same rank as $\boldsymbol{S}$. More specifically, any estimator is of rank p when $n \geq p$ and is of rank n when $p > n$.

Now, let $\widehat{\boldsymbol{\Sigma}}$ be an estimator of $\boldsymbol{\Sigma}$ based on $\boldsymbol{S}$ and $\boldsymbol{X}$ in (7.1), where $\widehat{\boldsymbol{\Sigma}} \in \mathbb{S}_{p,\nu}^{(+)}$. Since $\boldsymbol{\Sigma}^{-1}$ is positive definite, $\boldsymbol{\Sigma}^{-1}\widehat{\boldsymbol{\Sigma}}$ has ν nonzero eigenvalues and they are all positive. Let $\operatorname{Ch}(\boldsymbol{\Sigma}^{-1}\widehat{\boldsymbol{\Sigma}}) \in \mathbb{D}_\nu$ such that its diagonal elements consist of ν positive eigenvalues of $\boldsymbol{\Sigma}^{-1}\widehat{\boldsymbol{\Sigma}}$. The extended Stein loss is defined by

$$L_{ES}(\widehat{\boldsymbol{\Sigma}}, \boldsymbol{\Sigma}) = \operatorname{tr} [\operatorname{Ch}(\boldsymbol{\Sigma}^{-1}\widehat{\boldsymbol{\Sigma}})] - \log |\operatorname{Ch}(\boldsymbol{\Sigma}^{-1}\widehat{\boldsymbol{\Sigma}})| - \nu. \tag{7.3}$$

If $n \geq p$, L_{ES} is the same as the ordinary Stein loss (7.2). The accuracy of estimators is measured by the risk function $R_{ES}(\widehat{\boldsymbol{\Sigma}}, \boldsymbol{\Sigma}) = E[L_{ES}(\widehat{\boldsymbol{\Sigma}}, \boldsymbol{\Sigma})]$, where the expectation

E is taken with respect to the model (7.1). With the extended Stein loss (7.3) used, this chapter gives some dominance results unifying both cases of $n \geq p$ and $p > n$.

First in Sect. 7.2, we deal with the best scale invariant estimator that forms a scalar multiple of $\boldsymbol{S}$. Section 7.3 considers the class of triangular invariant estimators and gives a unified expression of the James-Stein (1961) type estimators for the $n \geq p$ and $p > n$ cases. Section 7.4 provides some orthogonally invariant estimators improving on the best scale invariant and the unified James-Stein-type estimators relative to the extended Stein loss (7.3). Section 7.5 gives alternative unified estimators using information on the mean statistic $\boldsymbol{X}$. In Sect. 7.6, we point out some relevant topics on decision-theoretic covariance estimation.

7.2 Scale Invariant Estimators

Recall that $\nu = n \wedge p$ and $\kappa = n \vee p$. Consider a simple class of estimators which forms a constant multiple of $\boldsymbol{S}$. The simple class is denoted by

$$\widehat{\boldsymbol{\Sigma}}_c = \widehat{\boldsymbol{\Sigma}}_c(\boldsymbol{S}) = c\boldsymbol{S}, \tag{7.4}$$

where c is a positive constant. The class (7.4) satisfies $\boldsymbol{P}\widehat{\boldsymbol{\Sigma}}_c(\boldsymbol{S})\boldsymbol{P}^\top = \widehat{\boldsymbol{\Sigma}}_c(\boldsymbol{P}\boldsymbol{S}\boldsymbol{P}^\top)$ for any $\boldsymbol{P} \in \mathbb{U}_p$, namely, $\widehat{\boldsymbol{\Sigma}}_c$ is invariant under the scale transformations $\boldsymbol{S} \to \boldsymbol{P}\boldsymbol{S}\boldsymbol{P}^\top$ and $\widehat{\boldsymbol{\Sigma}} \to \boldsymbol{P}\widehat{\boldsymbol{\Sigma}}\boldsymbol{P}^\top$ for any $\boldsymbol{P} \in \mathbb{U}_p$. The unbiased estimator of $\boldsymbol{\Sigma}$,

$$\widehat{\boldsymbol{\Sigma}}^{UB} = \frac{1}{n}\boldsymbol{S},$$

belongs to the class (7.4), but $\widehat{\boldsymbol{\Sigma}}^{UB}$ is not the best estimator among the class (7.4) relative to the extended Stein loss (7.3). The best estimator is given in the following proposition.

Proposition 7.1 *Among the class* (7.4), *the best estimator relative to the extended Stein loss* (7.3) *is given by*

$$\widehat{\boldsymbol{\Sigma}}^{BS} = \widehat{\boldsymbol{\Sigma}}_{c_0}$$

with $c_0 = 1/\kappa$. *Hence for* $p > n$, $\widehat{\boldsymbol{\Sigma}}^{BS} = \boldsymbol{S}/p$ *dominates* $\widehat{\boldsymbol{\Sigma}}^{UB} = \boldsymbol{S}/n$ *relative to the extended Stein loss* (7.3).

Proof Recall that $\boldsymbol{S} = \boldsymbol{Y}^\top\boldsymbol{Y}$ and $\boldsymbol{Y} \in \mathbb{R}^{n\times p}$. The positive eigenvalues of $\boldsymbol{\Sigma}^{-1}\boldsymbol{S}$ are identical to those of $\boldsymbol{Y}\boldsymbol{\Sigma}^{-1}\boldsymbol{Y}^\top$, so that the positive eigenvalues of $\boldsymbol{\Sigma}^{-1}\boldsymbol{S}$ are identical to those of the full-rank matrix

$$\begin{cases} \boldsymbol{\Sigma}^{-1}\boldsymbol{S} \ (\in \mathbb{R}^{p\times p}) & \text{for } n \geq p, \\ \boldsymbol{Y}\boldsymbol{\Sigma}^{-1}\boldsymbol{Y}^\top \ (\in \mathbb{S}_n^{(+)} \subset \mathbb{R}^{n\times n}) & \text{for } p > n. \end{cases}$$

Note that $\mathrm{tr}\,[\mathrm{Ch}(\boldsymbol{\Sigma}^{-1}\widehat{\boldsymbol{\Sigma}}_c)] = \mathrm{tr}\,\boldsymbol{\Sigma}^{-1}\widehat{\boldsymbol{\Sigma}}_c$. Since $\boldsymbol{\Sigma}^{-1}\boldsymbol{S}$ has ν positive eigenvalues with probability one, we obtain $|\mathrm{Ch}(c\boldsymbol{\Sigma}^{-1}\boldsymbol{S})| = c^{\nu}|\mathrm{Ch}(\boldsymbol{\Sigma}^{-1}\boldsymbol{S})|$. The risk of $\widehat{\boldsymbol{\Sigma}}_c$ with respect to the extended Stein loss (7.3) is expressed as

$$\begin{aligned} R_{ES}(\widehat{\boldsymbol{\Sigma}}_c, \boldsymbol{\Sigma}) &= nc\ \mathrm{tr}\,\boldsymbol{\Sigma}^{-1}\boldsymbol{\Sigma} - \nu \log c - E[\log|\mathrm{Ch}(\boldsymbol{\Sigma}^{-1}\boldsymbol{S})|] - \nu \\ &= npc - \nu \log c - E[\log|\mathrm{Ch}(\boldsymbol{\Sigma}^{-1}\boldsymbol{S})|] - \nu, \end{aligned}$$

which is minimized at $c = c_0$ with

$$c_0 = \frac{\nu}{np} = \frac{1}{\kappa}.$$

Thus the proof is complete. □

Denote $r_{\kappa,\nu} = E[\log|\mathrm{Ch}(\boldsymbol{\Sigma}^{-1}\boldsymbol{S})|]$. The risk of $\widehat{\boldsymbol{\Sigma}}^{BS}$ is

$$R_{ES}(\widehat{\boldsymbol{\Sigma}}^{BS}, \boldsymbol{\Sigma}) = \nu \log \kappa - r_{\kappa,\nu}. \tag{7.5}$$

Now, it follows that

$$|\mathrm{Ch}(\boldsymbol{\Sigma}^{-1}\boldsymbol{S})| = \begin{cases} |\boldsymbol{\Sigma}^{-1}\boldsymbol{Y}^\top\boldsymbol{Y}| & \text{for } n \ge p, \\ |\boldsymbol{Y}\boldsymbol{\Sigma}^{-1}\boldsymbol{Y}^\top| & \text{for } p > n, \end{cases}$$

and consequently

$$r_{\kappa,\nu} = \begin{cases} E[\log|\boldsymbol{Z}^\top\boldsymbol{Z}|] & \text{for } n \ge p, \\ E[\log|\boldsymbol{Z}\boldsymbol{Z}^\top|] & \text{for } p > n, \end{cases}$$

where $\boldsymbol{Z} \sim \mathcal{N}_{n\times p}(\boldsymbol{0}_{n\times p}, \boldsymbol{I}_n \otimes \boldsymbol{I}_p)$. Since $\boldsymbol{Z}^\top\boldsymbol{Z} \sim \mathcal{W}_p(n, \boldsymbol{I}_p)$ for $n \ge p$ and $\boldsymbol{Z}\boldsymbol{Z}^\top \sim \mathcal{W}_n(p, \boldsymbol{I}_n)$ for $p > n$, using Corollary 3.2 gives $r_{\kappa,\nu} = \sum_{i=1}^{\nu} E[\log s_i]$, where $s_i \sim \chi^2_{\kappa-i+1}$ for $i = 1, \ldots, \nu$. Denoting the digamma function by

$$\mathcal{F}(t) = \frac{\mathrm{d}}{\mathrm{d}t}\log\Gamma(t) = \frac{\Gamma'(t)}{\Gamma(t)},$$

we observe $E[\log s_i] = \mathcal{F}((\kappa - i + 1)/2) + \log 2$, so that

$$r_{\kappa,\nu} = \sum_{i=1}^{\nu} \mathcal{F}\left(\frac{\kappa - i + 1}{2}\right) + \nu \log 2.$$

Hence $r_{\kappa,\nu}$ is a constant and $\widehat{\boldsymbol{\Sigma}}^{BS}$ has a constant risk.

7.3 Triangular Invariant Estimators and the James-Stein Estimator

7.3.1 The James-Stein Estimator

As seen in Sect. 3.4, the Cholesky decomposition of $\boldsymbol{S}$ is written as

$$\boldsymbol{S} = \boldsymbol{T}\boldsymbol{T}^\top = \begin{pmatrix} \boldsymbol{T}_1 \\ \boldsymbol{T}_2 \end{pmatrix} (\boldsymbol{T}_1^\top, \boldsymbol{T}_2^\top),$$

where $\boldsymbol{T} = (\boldsymbol{T}_1^\top, \boldsymbol{T}_2^\top)^\top \in \mathbb{L}_{p,\nu}^{(+)}$, $\boldsymbol{T}_1 \in \mathbb{L}_\nu^{(+)}$ and $\boldsymbol{T}_2 \in \mathbb{R}^{(p-\nu)\times\nu}$. Define a class of estimators as

$$\widehat{\boldsymbol{\Sigma}}^T = \widehat{\boldsymbol{\Sigma}}^T(\boldsymbol{S}) = \boldsymbol{T}\boldsymbol{D}_\nu\boldsymbol{T}^\top, \tag{7.6}$$

where $\boldsymbol{D}_\nu = \mathrm{diag}\,(d_1, \ldots, d_\nu)$ and the d_i's are positive constants. The unbiased estimator $\widehat{\boldsymbol{\Sigma}}^{UB}$ and the best scale invariant estimator $\widehat{\boldsymbol{\Sigma}}^{BS}$ are members of the class (7.6).

The class (7.6) is invariant under the scale transformation with respect to the lower triangular group $\mathbb{L}_p^{(+)}$. Indeed, this can be verified as follows: Denote by $\boldsymbol{T}_*\boldsymbol{T}_*^\top$ the Cholesky decomposition of $\boldsymbol{L}\boldsymbol{S}\boldsymbol{L}^\top$ for $\boldsymbol{L} \in \mathbb{L}_p^{(+)}$. It is observed that $\boldsymbol{L}\boldsymbol{S}\boldsymbol{L}^\top = \boldsymbol{L}\boldsymbol{T}\boldsymbol{T}^\top\boldsymbol{L}^\top$ and $\boldsymbol{L}\boldsymbol{T} \in \mathbb{L}_{p,\nu}^{(+)}$. As discussed in the beginning of Sect. 3.4, the Cholesky decomposition of a symmetric positive semi-definite matrix $\boldsymbol{S}$ is unique. Thus, we obtain $\boldsymbol{T}_* = \boldsymbol{L}\boldsymbol{T}$, so that

$$\widehat{\boldsymbol{\Sigma}}^T(\boldsymbol{L}\boldsymbol{S}\boldsymbol{L}^\top) = \boldsymbol{T}_*\boldsymbol{D}_\nu\boldsymbol{T}_*^\top = \boldsymbol{L}\boldsymbol{T}\boldsymbol{D}_\nu\boldsymbol{T}^\top\boldsymbol{L}^\top = \boldsymbol{L}\widehat{\boldsymbol{\Sigma}}^T(\boldsymbol{S})\boldsymbol{L}^\top.$$

Here $\widehat{\boldsymbol{\Sigma}}^T$ is named triangular invariant estimator. We will now investigate the risk function of $\widehat{\boldsymbol{\Sigma}}^T$. The Cholesky decomposition of $\boldsymbol{\Sigma}$ is expressed as $\boldsymbol{\Sigma} = \boldsymbol{\Xi}\boldsymbol{\Xi}^\top$, where $\boldsymbol{\Xi} \in \mathbb{L}_p^{(+)}$. Let $\boldsymbol{U} = \boldsymbol{\Xi}^{-1}\boldsymbol{T}$. Then

$$\begin{aligned} E[\mathrm{tr}\,[\mathrm{Ch}(\boldsymbol{\Sigma}^{-1}\widehat{\boldsymbol{\Sigma}}^T)]] &= E[\mathrm{tr}\,\boldsymbol{D}_\nu\boldsymbol{T}^\top\boldsymbol{\Sigma}^{-1}\boldsymbol{T}] \\ &= E[\mathrm{tr}\,\boldsymbol{D}_\nu(\boldsymbol{\Xi}^{-1}\boldsymbol{T})^\top\boldsymbol{\Xi}^{-1}\boldsymbol{T}] \\ &= E[\mathrm{tr}\,\boldsymbol{D}_\nu\boldsymbol{U}^\top\boldsymbol{U}]. \end{aligned} \tag{7.7}$$

The distributions of nonzero elements of $\boldsymbol{U}$ are given in Corollary 3.2. In the $p > n$ case, we partition $\boldsymbol{U}$ as $\boldsymbol{U} = (u_{ij}) = (\boldsymbol{U}_1^\top, \boldsymbol{U}_2^\top)^\top$, where $\boldsymbol{U}_1 \in \mathbb{L}_n^{(+)}$. Since $\boldsymbol{U}_2 \sim \mathcal{N}_{(p-n)\times n}(\boldsymbol{0}_{(p-n)\times n}, \boldsymbol{I}_{(p-n)} \otimes \boldsymbol{I}_n)$, Corollary 3.1 leads to $E[\boldsymbol{U}_2^\top\boldsymbol{U}_2] = (p-n)\boldsymbol{I}_n$. For $i = 1, \ldots, n$, the i-th diagonal element of $E[\boldsymbol{U}_1^\top\boldsymbol{U}_1]$ is

$$\begin{aligned} \sum_{j=i}^{n} E[u_{ji}^2] &= E[u_{ii}^2] + \sum_{j>i}^{n} E[u_{ji}^2] \\ &= (n-i+1) + (n-i) = 2n - 2i + 1, \end{aligned}$$

so that

$$E[\operatorname{tr} \boldsymbol{D}_n \boldsymbol{U}^\top \boldsymbol{U}] = \operatorname{tr} \boldsymbol{D}_n E[\boldsymbol{U}_1^\top \boldsymbol{U}_1] + \operatorname{tr} \boldsymbol{D}_n E[\boldsymbol{U}_2^\top \boldsymbol{U}_2]$$
$$= \sum_{i=1}^{n} \{(2n - 2i + 1)d_i + (p - n)d_i\}$$
$$= \sum_{i=1}^{n} (n + p - 2i + 1)d_i. \tag{7.8}$$

When $n \geq p$, it follows that

$$E[\operatorname{tr} \boldsymbol{D}_p \boldsymbol{U}^\top \boldsymbol{U}] = \sum_{i=1}^{p} \sum_{j=i}^{p} E[d_i u_{ji}^2] = \sum_{i=1}^{p} (n + p - 2i + 1)d_i. \tag{7.9}$$

Combining (7.7), (7.8) and (7.9) gives

$$E[\operatorname{tr} [\operatorname{Ch}(\boldsymbol{\Sigma}^{-1} \widehat{\boldsymbol{\Sigma}}^T)]] = \sum_{i=1}^{\nu} (n + p - 2i + 1)d_i. \tag{7.10}$$

It is seen that $\boldsymbol{\Sigma}^{-1} \widehat{\boldsymbol{\Sigma}}^T$ has the same positive eigenvalues as $\boldsymbol{D}_\nu \boldsymbol{T}^\top \boldsymbol{\Sigma}^{-1} \boldsymbol{T}$, implying that

$$|\operatorname{Ch}(\boldsymbol{\Sigma}^{-1} \widehat{\boldsymbol{\Sigma}}^T)| = |\boldsymbol{D}_\nu \boldsymbol{T}^\top \boldsymbol{\Sigma}^{-1} \boldsymbol{T}|.$$

Since $\boldsymbol{T}^\top \boldsymbol{\Sigma}^{-1} \boldsymbol{T} \in \mathbb{S}_\nu^{(+)}$, it follows that

$$E[\log |\operatorname{Ch}(\boldsymbol{\Sigma}^{-1} \widehat{\boldsymbol{\Sigma}}^T)|] = \log |\boldsymbol{D}_\nu| + E[\log |\boldsymbol{T}^\top \boldsymbol{\Sigma}^{-1} \boldsymbol{T}|] = \sum_{i=1}^{\nu} \log d_i + r_{\kappa,\nu}, \tag{7.11}$$

where $r_{\kappa,\nu}$ is the same as in (7.5). Using (7.10) and (7.11), we can write the risk of $\widehat{\boldsymbol{\Sigma}}^T$ under the extended Stein loss (7.3) as

$$R_{ES}(\widehat{\boldsymbol{\Sigma}}^T, \boldsymbol{\Sigma}) = \sum_{i=1}^{\nu} \{(n + p - 2i + 1)d_i - \log d_i\} - r_{\kappa,\nu} - \nu.$$

Hence the triangular invariant estimator $\widehat{\boldsymbol{\Sigma}}^T$ has a constant risk.

Clearly, the d_i's minimizing the risk $R_{ES}(\widehat{\boldsymbol{\Sigma}}^T, \boldsymbol{\Sigma})$ are given by

$$d_i^{JS} = \frac{1}{n + p - 2i + 1}$$

for $i = 1, \ldots, \nu$. Thus the best triangular invariant estimator can be expressed as

$$\widehat{\boldsymbol{\Sigma}}^{JS} = \boldsymbol{T}\boldsymbol{D}_{\nu}^{JS}\boldsymbol{T}^{\top}, \tag{7.12}$$

where $\boldsymbol{D}_{\nu}^{JS} = \mathrm{diag}\,(d_1^{JS}, \ldots, d_{\nu}^{JS})$, which is named the James-Stein (1961) estimator. Since $\widehat{\boldsymbol{\Sigma}}^{BS}$ belongs to the class (7.6), $\widehat{\boldsymbol{\Sigma}}^{JS}$ dominates $\widehat{\boldsymbol{\Sigma}}^{BS}$ relative to the extended Stein loss (7.3). In fact, $\widehat{\boldsymbol{\Sigma}}^{JS}$ has the constant risk

$$R_{ES}(\widehat{\boldsymbol{\Sigma}}^{JS}, \boldsymbol{\Sigma}) = \sum_{i=1}^{\nu} \log(n + p - 2i + 1) - r_{\kappa,\nu}, \tag{7.13}$$

which implies by (7.5) that

$$R_{ES}(\widehat{\boldsymbol{\Sigma}}^{JS}, \boldsymbol{\Sigma}) - R_{ES}(\widehat{\boldsymbol{\Sigma}}^{BS}, \boldsymbol{\Sigma}) = \sum_{i=1}^{\nu} \log(n + p - 2i + 1) - \nu \log \kappa < 0,$$

where the inequality follows immediately from concavity of the logarithmic function.

The abovementioned can be summarized as follows.

Proposition 7.2 *The James-Stein estimator $\widehat{\boldsymbol{\Sigma}}^{JS}$, namely, the best triangular invariant estimator dominates the best scale invariant estimator $\widehat{\boldsymbol{\Sigma}}^{BS}$ relative to the extended Stein loss* (7.3).

As pointed out by Stein (1956) and James and Stein (1961), $\widehat{\boldsymbol{\Sigma}}^{JS}$ is minimax when $n \geq p$. The proof of minimaxity comes from the invariance approach. A general theory of the invariance approach was studied in Kiefer (1957). For proving minimaxity of a specific estimator, the least favorable prior approach are also well known (Strawderman, 2000). See Tsukuma and Kubokawa (2015) for the minimaxity proof of $\widehat{\boldsymbol{\Sigma}}^{JS}$ by using the least favorable prior approach.

7.3.2 *Improvement Using a Subgroup Invariance*

In the literature, various estimators have been proposed for improving the James-Stein estimator $\widehat{\boldsymbol{\Sigma}}^{JS}$ in (7.12). Here we introduce an invariant estimator under the commutator subgroup of $\mathbb{L}_p^{(+)}$.

For two elements $\boldsymbol{A}$ and $\boldsymbol{B}$ of the group $\mathbb{L}_p^{(+)}$, the commutator of $\boldsymbol{A}$ and $\boldsymbol{B}$ is defined by $\boldsymbol{A}^{-1}\boldsymbol{B}^{-1}\boldsymbol{A}\boldsymbol{B}$. The commutator subgroup of $\mathbb{L}_p^{(+)}$ is generated by all the commutators of $\mathbb{L}_p^{(+)}$ and coincides with $\mathbb{L}_p^{(1)}$, where $\mathbb{L}_p^{(1)}$ consists of all $p \times p$ lower triangular matrices with ones on the diagonal.

Let $\boldsymbol{S} = \boldsymbol{T}_1\boldsymbol{T}_0\boldsymbol{T}_1^{\top}$, where $\boldsymbol{T}_0$ and $\boldsymbol{T}_1$ are, respectively, unique elements of $\mathbb{D}_{\nu}$ and $\mathbb{L}_{p,\nu}^{(1)}$. Note that, when $n \geq p$, $\boldsymbol{T}_1\boldsymbol{T}_0\boldsymbol{T}_1^{\top}$ is the LDL$^{\top}$ decomposition of $\boldsymbol{S}$. Here we define a class of estimators as

$$\widehat{\boldsymbol{\Sigma}}^{I} = \widehat{\boldsymbol{\Sigma}}^{I}(\boldsymbol{T}_0, \boldsymbol{T}_1) = \boldsymbol{T}_1\boldsymbol{\Phi}(\boldsymbol{T}_0)\boldsymbol{T}_1^{\top}, \tag{7.14}$$

where $\boldsymbol{\Phi}(\boldsymbol{T}_0) \in \mathbb{D}_\nu$ and each diagonal element of $\boldsymbol{\Phi}(\boldsymbol{T}_0)$ is an absolutely continuous function of $\boldsymbol{T}_0$. The class (7.14) is invariant under the transformations $\boldsymbol{S} \to \boldsymbol{A}\boldsymbol{S}\boldsymbol{A}^\top$ and $\widehat{\boldsymbol{\Sigma}} \to \boldsymbol{A}\widehat{\boldsymbol{\Sigma}}\boldsymbol{A}^\top$ for any $\boldsymbol{A} \in \mathbb{L}_p^{(1)}$.

The risk of the class (7.14) can be expressed as follows.

Theorem 7.1 *Denote* $\boldsymbol{T}_0 = \mathrm{diag}\,(t_1, \ldots, t_\nu)$ *and* $\boldsymbol{\Phi}(\boldsymbol{T}_0) = \mathrm{diag}\,(\phi_1, \ldots, \phi_\nu)$. *Then the risk function of* $\widehat{\boldsymbol{\Sigma}}^I$ *with respect to the extended Stein loss (7.3) is expressed by*

$$R_{ES}(\widehat{\boldsymbol{\Sigma}}^I, \boldsymbol{\Sigma}) = E\bigg[\sum_{i=1}^{\nu}\bigg\{(n+p-2i-1)\frac{\phi_i}{t_i} + 2\frac{\partial \phi_i}{\partial t_i} - \log\frac{\phi_i}{t_i}\bigg\}\bigg] - r_{\kappa,\nu} - \nu,$$

where $r_{\kappa,\nu}$ *is given by (7.5).*

Proof It is observed that

$$\begin{aligned}\log|\mathrm{Ch}(\boldsymbol{\Sigma}^{-1}\widehat{\boldsymbol{\Sigma}}^I)| &= \log|\mathrm{Ch}(\boldsymbol{T}_1^\top\boldsymbol{\Sigma}^{-1}\boldsymbol{T}_1\boldsymbol{T}_0\boldsymbol{T}_0^{-1}\boldsymbol{\Phi}(\boldsymbol{T}_0))| \\ &= \log|\mathrm{Ch}(\boldsymbol{T}_1^\top\boldsymbol{\Sigma}^{-1}\boldsymbol{T}_1\boldsymbol{T}_0)| + \log|\mathrm{Ch}(\boldsymbol{T}_0^{-1}\boldsymbol{\Phi}(\boldsymbol{T}_0))| \\ &= \log|\mathrm{Ch}(\boldsymbol{\Sigma}^{-1}\boldsymbol{S})| + \sum_{i=1}^{\nu}\log\frac{\phi_i}{t_i},\end{aligned}$$

so that

$$E[\log|\mathrm{Ch}(\boldsymbol{\Sigma}^{-1}\widehat{\boldsymbol{\Sigma}}^I)|] = E\bigg[\sum_{i=1}^{\nu}\log\frac{\phi_i}{t_i}\bigg] + r_{\kappa,\nu}.$$

Thus,

$$\begin{aligned}R_{ES}(\widehat{\boldsymbol{\Sigma}}^I, \boldsymbol{\Sigma}) &= E[\mathrm{tr}\,\boldsymbol{\Sigma}^{-1}\boldsymbol{T}_1\boldsymbol{\Phi}(\boldsymbol{T}_0)\boldsymbol{T}_1^\top - \log|\mathrm{Ch}(\boldsymbol{\Sigma}^{-1}\boldsymbol{T}_1\boldsymbol{\Phi}(\boldsymbol{T}_0)\boldsymbol{T}_1^\top)| - \nu] \\ &= E\bigg[\mathrm{tr}\,\boldsymbol{\Sigma}^{-1}\boldsymbol{T}_1\boldsymbol{\Phi}(\boldsymbol{T}_0)\boldsymbol{T}_1^\top - \sum_{i=1}^{\nu}\log\frac{\phi_i}{t_i}\bigg] - r_{\kappa,\nu} - \nu. \qquad (7.15)\end{aligned}$$

Denote by $\boldsymbol{\Sigma}^{-1} = \boldsymbol{\Gamma}^\top\boldsymbol{\Sigma}_0^{-1}\boldsymbol{\Gamma}$ the LDL$^\top$ decomposition of $\boldsymbol{\Sigma}^{-1}$, where $\boldsymbol{\Sigma}_0 = \mathrm{diag}\,(\sigma_1^2, \ldots, \sigma_p^2)$ and $\boldsymbol{\Gamma}$ are, respectively, unique elements of $\mathbb{D}_p$ and $\mathbb{L}_p^{(1)}$. Making the transformation $\boldsymbol{U} = (u_{ij}) = \boldsymbol{\Gamma}\boldsymbol{T}_1$ $(\in \mathbb{L}_{p,\nu}^{(1)})$ yields

$$\begin{aligned}E[\mathrm{tr}\,\boldsymbol{\Sigma}^{-1}\widehat{\boldsymbol{\Sigma}}^I] = E[\mathrm{tr}\,\boldsymbol{\Sigma}_0^{-1}\boldsymbol{U}\boldsymbol{\Phi}(\boldsymbol{T}_0)\boldsymbol{U}^\top] &= E\bigg[\sum_{i=1}^{\nu}\{\boldsymbol{U}^\top\boldsymbol{\Sigma}_0^{-1}\boldsymbol{U}\}_{ii}\phi_i\bigg] \\ &= E\bigg[\sum_{i=1}^{\nu}\phi_i\sum_{j=i}^{p}\frac{u_{ji}^2}{\sigma_j^2}\bigg].\end{aligned}$$

Using Proposition 3.10 with some manipulation, we can see that $t_i \sim \sigma_i^2 \chi^2_{n-i+1}$ for $i = 1, \dots, \nu$ and $u_{ji}|t_i \sim \mathcal{N}(0, (t_i/\sigma_j^2)^{-1})$ for $j > i$. Noting that $\boldsymbol{U} \in \mathbb{L}^{(1)}_{p,\nu}$, namely, $u_{ii} = 1$, we obtain

$$E[\operatorname{tr} \boldsymbol{\Sigma}^{-1}\widehat{\boldsymbol{\Sigma}}^I] = E\Big[\sum_{i=1}^{\nu} \phi_i(1/\sigma_i^2 + (p-i)/t_i)\Big],$$

which implies by the chi-square identity (5.4) that

$$E[\operatorname{tr} \boldsymbol{\Sigma}^{-1}\widehat{\boldsymbol{\Sigma}}^I] = E\Big[\sum_{i=1}^{\nu}\Big\{(n+p-2i-1)\frac{\phi_i}{t_i} + 2\frac{\partial \phi_i}{\partial t_i}\Big\}\Big]. \tag{7.16}$$

Hence combining (7.15) and (7.16) completes the proof. □

The James-Stein estimator $\widehat{\boldsymbol{\Sigma}}^{JS}$ belongs to the class (7.14). Using Theorem 7.1 with $\phi_i^{JS} = d_i^{JS} t_i$, we can obtain the same expression for risk of $\widehat{\boldsymbol{\Sigma}}^{JS}$ as in (7.13).

Next, we provide an improved estimator on $\widehat{\boldsymbol{\Sigma}}^{JS}$. Let $\boldsymbol{\Phi}^M(\boldsymbol{T}_0) = \operatorname{diag}(\phi_1^M, \dots, \phi_\nu^M)$ with

$$\phi_i^M = d_i^{JS} t_i - \frac{(t_i \log t_i) g(w)}{b+w}, \qquad w = \sum_{i=1}^{\nu} (\log t_i)^2,$$

where b is a suitable constant and $g(w)$ is a differentiable function of w.

Proposition 7.3 *Suppose* $\nu \ge 3$ *and* $b \ge 144(\nu-2)^2/\{25(n+p-1)^2\}$. *If* $g(w)$ *is nondecreasing in* w *and* $0 < g(w) \le 12(\nu-2)/\{5(n+p-1)^2\}$, *then*

$$\widehat{\boldsymbol{\Sigma}}^M = \widehat{\boldsymbol{\Sigma}}^M(\boldsymbol{T}_0, \boldsymbol{T}_1) = \boldsymbol{T}_1 \boldsymbol{\Phi}^M(\boldsymbol{T}_0)\boldsymbol{T}_1^\top$$

dominates $\widehat{\boldsymbol{\Sigma}}^{JS}$ *relative to the extended Stein loss (7.3).*

Proof This dominance result is proved along the same arguments as in Dey and Srinivasan (1985). For details, see Tsukuma (2014a). □

Proposition 7.3 implies that the best invariant estimator $\widehat{\boldsymbol{\Sigma}}^{JS}$ under $\mathbb{L}^{(+)}_p$ is dominated by the invariant estimator $\widehat{\boldsymbol{\Sigma}}^M$ under the commutator subgroup of $\mathbb{L}^{(+)}_p$, namely, under $\mathbb{L}^{(1)}_p$. Since the lower triangular group $\mathbb{L}^{(+)}_p$ is solvable, $\mathbb{L}^{(1)}_p$ also has a commutator subgroup. It is still not known whether there exists an invariant estimator under the commutator subgroup of $\mathbb{L}^{(1)}_p$ which dominates $\widehat{\boldsymbol{\Sigma}}^M$.

7.4 Orthogonally Invariant Estimators

7.4.1 Class of Orthogonally Invariant Estimators

The triangular invariant estimator $\widehat{\boldsymbol{\Sigma}}^T$ in (7.6) depends on the coordinate system. This fact causes inadmissibility of the James-Stein estimator $\widehat{\boldsymbol{\Sigma}}^{JS}$ in (7.12). For example, the inadmissibility can be shown by using the same arguments as in Stein (1956): Let $\boldsymbol{P}$ be a $p \times p$ unit anti-diagonal matrix of the form

$$\boldsymbol{P} = \begin{pmatrix} 0 & & 1 \\ & \cdot^{\cdot^{\cdot}} & \\ 1 & & 0 \end{pmatrix},$$

which is symmetric and orthogonal. Denote $\boldsymbol{Y} = (\boldsymbol{y}_1, \ldots, \boldsymbol{y}_n)^\top \in \mathbb{R}^{n \times p}$. Note that, for each $i = 1, \ldots, n$, $\boldsymbol{P}\boldsymbol{y}_i$ is a p-dimensional vector obtained from $\boldsymbol{y}_i$ by reversing the order of coordinates. Define the Cholesky decomposition of $\boldsymbol{PSP} = \boldsymbol{PY}^\top \boldsymbol{YP}$ as $\boldsymbol{T}_*\boldsymbol{T}_*^\top$, where $\boldsymbol{T}_* \in \mathbb{L}_{p,\nu}^{(+)}$ and $\boldsymbol{T}_*\boldsymbol{T}_*^\top$ is not the same as the Cholesky decomposition of $\boldsymbol{S}$ because of its uniqueness. Let $\widehat{\boldsymbol{\Sigma}}^U = \boldsymbol{T}_*\boldsymbol{D}_\nu^{JS}\boldsymbol{T}_*$, which is the best triangular invariant estimator of $\boldsymbol{P\Sigma P}$. Here $\boldsymbol{P}\widehat{\boldsymbol{\Sigma}}^U\boldsymbol{P}$ becomes an estimator of $\boldsymbol{\Sigma}$ and has the same risk as $\widehat{\boldsymbol{\Sigma}}^{JS}$. From the convexity of the extended Stein loss (7.3), it is easily proved that $\widehat{\boldsymbol{\Sigma}}^{JS}$ is dominated by a combination estimator $(\widehat{\boldsymbol{\Sigma}}^{JS} + \boldsymbol{P}\widehat{\boldsymbol{\Sigma}}^U\boldsymbol{P})/2$.

In this section, we will consider a general class of estimators not depending on the coordinate system and aim to find better estimators dominating $\widehat{\boldsymbol{\Sigma}}^{JS}$ and $\widehat{\boldsymbol{\Sigma}}^{BS}$ relative to the extended Stein loss (7.3). Write the eigenvalue decomposition of $\boldsymbol{S}$ as

$$\boldsymbol{S} = \boldsymbol{HLH}^\top,$$

where $\boldsymbol{L} = \mathrm{diag}\,(\ell_1, \ldots, \ell_\nu) \in \mathbb{D}_\nu^{(\geq 0)}$ and $\boldsymbol{H} \in \mathbb{V}_{p,\nu}$. The general class of estimators is defined by

$$\widehat{\boldsymbol{\Sigma}}^O = \widehat{\boldsymbol{\Sigma}}^O(\boldsymbol{S}) = \boldsymbol{H}\,\mathrm{diag}\,(\ell_1\phi_1(\boldsymbol{L}), \ldots, \ell_\nu\phi_\nu(\boldsymbol{L}))\boldsymbol{H}^\top = \boldsymbol{HL\Phi}(\boldsymbol{L})\boldsymbol{H}^\top,$$

where $\boldsymbol{\Phi}(\boldsymbol{L}) = \mathrm{diag}\,(\phi_1(\boldsymbol{L}), \ldots, \phi_\nu(\boldsymbol{L}))$ and the $\phi_i(\boldsymbol{L})$'s are absolutely continuous functions of $\boldsymbol{L}$. The class $\widehat{\boldsymbol{\Sigma}}^O$ is not only invariant with respect to exchanging coordinates, but also, more generally, orthogonally invariant in the sense that it satisfies $\boldsymbol{O}\widehat{\boldsymbol{\Sigma}}^O(\boldsymbol{S})\boldsymbol{O}^\top = \widehat{\boldsymbol{\Sigma}}^O(\boldsymbol{OSO}^\top)$ for any $\boldsymbol{O} \in \mathbb{O}_p$.

7.4.2 Unbiased Risk Estimate

Here, we will derive an unbiased risk estimate for orthogonally invariant estimators $\widehat{\boldsymbol{\Sigma}}^O$. Abbreviate $\phi_i(\boldsymbol{L})$ by ϕ_i. Since

$$H = HH^\top H = SS^+H = Y^\top YS^+H$$

with $Y \sim \mathcal{N}_{n\times p}(\mathbf{0}_{n\times p}, I_n \otimes \Sigma)$, it follows from Theorem 5.1 and Lemma 5.3 that

$$\begin{aligned} E[\operatorname{tr}[\operatorname{Ch}(\Sigma^{-1}\widehat{\Sigma}^O)]] &= E[\operatorname{tr}\Sigma^{-1}HL\Phi(L)H^\top] \\ &= E[\operatorname{tr}\nabla_Y^\top YS^+HL\Phi(L)H^\top] \\ &= E\Bigg[\sum_{i=1}^{\nu}\Bigg\{(|n-p|+1)\phi_i + 2\ell_i\frac{\partial\phi_i}{\partial\ell_i} + 2\sum_{j>i}^{\nu}\frac{\ell_i\phi_i - \ell_j\phi_j}{\ell_i-\ell_j}\Bigg\}\Bigg]. \end{aligned} \tag{7.17}$$

Note that $|\operatorname{Ch}(\Sigma^{-1}\widehat{\Sigma}^O)| = |H^\top\Sigma^{-1}HL|\cdot|\Phi(L)| = |\operatorname{Ch}(\Sigma^{-1}S)|\prod_{i=1}^{\nu}\phi_i$. The risk of $\widehat{\Sigma}^O$ becomes

$$\begin{aligned} R_{ES}(\widehat{\Sigma}^O, \Sigma) &= E[\operatorname{tr}\Sigma^{-1}\widehat{\Sigma}^O - \log|\operatorname{Ch}(\Sigma^{-1}\widehat{\Sigma}^O)| - \nu] \\ &= E\Bigg[\sum_{i=1}^{\nu}\Bigg\{(|n-p|+1)\phi_i + 2\ell_i\frac{\partial\phi_i}{\partial\ell_i} + 2\sum_{j>i}^{\nu}\frac{\ell_i\phi_i - \ell_j\phi_j}{\ell_i-\ell_j} - \log\phi_i\Bigg\}\Bigg] \\ &\quad - r_{K,\nu} - \nu. \end{aligned}$$

Hence, we obtain the unbiased risk estimate for $\widehat{\Sigma}^O$,

$$\widehat{R}_{ES}(\widehat{\Sigma}^O) = \sum_{i=1}^{\nu}\Bigg\{(|n-p|+1)\phi_i + 2\ell_i\frac{\partial\phi_i}{\partial\ell_i} + 2\sum_{j>i}^{\nu}\frac{\ell_i\phi_i - \ell_j\phi_j}{\ell_i-\ell_j} - \log\phi_i\Bigg\} - r_{K,\nu} - \nu. \tag{7.18}$$

Comparing (7.5), or (7.13), with (7.18) gives a sufficient condition that $\widehat{\Sigma}^O$ dominates $\widehat{\Sigma}^{BS}$, or $\widehat{\Sigma}^{JS}$, relative to the extended Stein loss (7.3). For example, we denote the difference between $\widehat{R}_{ES}(\widehat{\Sigma}^O)$ and (7.13) by

$$\begin{aligned} \widehat{\Delta}(\widehat{\Sigma}^O) &= \widehat{R}_{ES}(\widehat{\Sigma}^O) - R_{ES}(\widehat{\Sigma}^{JS}, \Sigma) \\ &= \sum_{i=1}^{\nu}\Bigg\{(|n-p|+1)\phi_i + 2\ell_i\frac{\partial\phi_i}{\partial\ell_i} + 2\sum_{j>i}^{\nu}\frac{\ell_i\phi_i - \ell_j\phi_j}{\ell_i-\ell_j} - \log\phi_i\Bigg\} \\ &\quad + \sum_{i=1}^{\nu}\log d_i^{JS} - \nu, \end{aligned} \tag{7.19}$$

implying that if $\widehat{\Delta}(\widehat{\Sigma}^O) \le 0$ for every $L \in \mathbb{D}_\nu^{(\ge 0)}$ then $\widehat{\Sigma}^O$ dominates $\widehat{\Sigma}^{JS}$.

7.4.3 Examples

7.4.3.1 Haff's Empirical Bayes Estimator

When $n \geq p$, Haff (1980) considered the empirical Bayes estimation of $\boldsymbol{\Sigma}$. For the sake of simplicity, let a prior distribution of $\boldsymbol{\Sigma}^{-1}$ be $\mathcal{W}_p(p+1, \gamma^{-1}\boldsymbol{I}_p)$, where γ is an unknown hyperparameter. The resulting posterior distribution of $\boldsymbol{\Sigma}^{-1}$ given $\boldsymbol{S}$ is $\boldsymbol{\Sigma}^{-1}|\boldsymbol{S} \sim \mathcal{W}_p(n+p+1, (\boldsymbol{S}+\gamma\boldsymbol{I}_p)^{-1})$, so that the posterior mean of $\boldsymbol{\Sigma}$ is $E[\boldsymbol{\Sigma}|\boldsymbol{S}] = n^{-1}(\boldsymbol{S}+\gamma\boldsymbol{I}_p)$, where this expectation will be explained in Sect. 7.6.4. The hyperparameter γ is estimated from the marginal density of $\boldsymbol{S}$ proportional to

$$\gamma^{p(p+1)/2}|\boldsymbol{S}|^{(n-p-1)/2}|\boldsymbol{S}+\gamma\boldsymbol{I}_p|^{-(n+p+1)/2}.$$

The log-likelihood function with ignoring a constant has the form

$$l(\gamma|\boldsymbol{S}) = \frac{p(p+1)}{2}\log\gamma - \frac{n+p+1}{2}\log|\boldsymbol{I}_p + \gamma\boldsymbol{S}^{-1}|.$$

The first order approximation of $\log|\boldsymbol{I}_p + \gamma\boldsymbol{S}^{-1}|$ is $\gamma \operatorname{tr}\boldsymbol{S}^{-1}$, so that the log-likelihood function can be approximated as

$$l(\gamma|\boldsymbol{S}) \approx \frac{p(p+1)}{2}\log\gamma - \frac{n+p+1}{2}\gamma\operatorname{tr}\boldsymbol{S}^{-1},$$

which attains a maximum at

$$\widehat{\gamma} = \frac{p(p+1)}{n+p+1}\frac{1}{\operatorname{tr}\boldsymbol{S}^{-1}}.$$

The estimate $\widehat{\gamma}$ is an approximated maximum likelihood estimate for γ. Thus we obtain an empirical Bayes estimator of the form

$$\widehat{\boldsymbol{\Sigma}}^{EB} = \frac{1}{n}(\boldsymbol{S}+\widehat{\gamma}\boldsymbol{I}_p) = \frac{1}{n}\left(\boldsymbol{S} + \frac{p(p+1)}{n+p+1}\frac{1}{\operatorname{tr}\boldsymbol{S}^{-1}}\boldsymbol{I}_p\right).$$

Haff (1980) defined a general class of empirical Bayes estimators and gave some dominance results.

Here, taking into account both the cases of $n \geq p$ and $p > n$, we define a Haff type estimator as

$$\widehat{\boldsymbol{\Sigma}}^{HF} = \widehat{\boldsymbol{\Sigma}}^{BS} + \frac{a}{\kappa\operatorname{tr}\boldsymbol{S}^{+}}\boldsymbol{S}\boldsymbol{S}^{+},$$

where a is a positive constant. Since $\operatorname{tr}\boldsymbol{S}^{+} = \operatorname{tr}\boldsymbol{L}^{-1}$ and $\boldsymbol{S}\boldsymbol{S}^{+} = \boldsymbol{H}\boldsymbol{H}^\top$ for $\boldsymbol{S} = \boldsymbol{H}\boldsymbol{L}\boldsymbol{H}^\top$, the Haff estimator can be expressed as

$$\widehat{\boldsymbol{\Sigma}}^{HF} = \boldsymbol{H}\boldsymbol{L}\boldsymbol{\Phi}^{HF}(\boldsymbol{L})\boldsymbol{H}^\top, \quad \boldsymbol{\Phi}^{HF}(\boldsymbol{L}) = \frac{1}{\kappa}\Big(\boldsymbol{I}_\nu + \frac{a}{\operatorname{tr}\boldsymbol{L}^{-1}}\boldsymbol{L}^{-1}\Big).$$

Proposition 7.4 *If* $0 < a \le 2(\nu-1)/(|n-p|+1)$*, then* $\widehat{\boldsymbol{\Sigma}}^{HF}$ *dominates* $\widehat{\boldsymbol{\Sigma}}^{BS}$ *relative to the extended Stein loss* (7.3).

Proof For $i = 1, \dots, \nu$, let $\phi_i^{HF} = \kappa^{-1}(1 + a\ell_i^{-1}/\operatorname{tr}\boldsymbol{L}^{-1})$. Note that

$$\sum_{i=1}^{\nu} \ell_i \frac{\partial \phi_i^{HF}}{\partial \ell_i} = \frac{a}{\kappa}\Big(-1 + \frac{\operatorname{tr}\boldsymbol{L}^{-2}}{(\operatorname{tr}\boldsymbol{L}^{-1})^2}\Big) \le 0,$$

so that, by (7.18),

$$\begin{aligned}\widehat{R}_{ES}(\widehat{\boldsymbol{\Sigma}}^{HF}) &= \sum_{i=1}^{\nu}\Big\{(|n-p|+1)\phi_i^{HF} + 2\ell_i\frac{\partial\phi_i^{HF}}{\partial\ell_i} + 2\sum_{j>i}^{\nu}\frac{\ell_i\phi_i^{HF} - \ell_j\phi_j^{HF}}{\ell_i - \ell_j} \\ &\quad - \log\phi_i^{HF}\Big\} - r_{\kappa,\nu} - \nu \\ &\le \widehat{R}_{ES}(\widehat{\boldsymbol{\Sigma}}^{BS}) + (|n-p|+1)\frac{a}{\kappa} - \sum_{i=1}^{\nu}\log(1 + a\ell_i^{-1}/\operatorname{tr}\boldsymbol{L}^{-1}).\end{aligned}$$

Since $\log(1+x) \ge 2x/(2+x)$ for $x \ge 0$, it holds that

$$\begin{aligned}\sum_{i=1}^{\nu}\log(1 + a\ell_i^{-1}/\operatorname{tr}\boldsymbol{L}^{-1}) &\ge \sum_{i=1}^{\nu}\frac{2a\ell_i^{-1}/\operatorname{tr}\boldsymbol{L}^{-1}}{2 + a\ell_i^{-1}/\operatorname{tr}\boldsymbol{L}^{-1}} \\ &\ge \sum_{i=1}^{\nu}\frac{2a\ell_i^{-1}/\operatorname{tr}\boldsymbol{L}^{-1}}{2+a} = \frac{2a}{2+a},\end{aligned}$$

which yields

$$\widehat{R}_{ES}(\widehat{\boldsymbol{\Sigma}}^{HF}) - \widehat{R}_{ES}(\widehat{\boldsymbol{\Sigma}}^{BS}) \le (|n-p|+1)\frac{a}{\kappa} - \frac{2a}{2+a} = \frac{a}{2+a}\{(|n-p|+1)a - 2(\nu-1)\}.$$

Hence we complete the proof. □

7.4.3.2 The Efron-Morris-Dey Shrinkage Estimator

Since $\widehat{\boldsymbol{\Sigma}}^{HF} \succeq \widehat{\boldsymbol{\Sigma}}^{BS}$, the Haff estimator $\widehat{\boldsymbol{\Sigma}}^{HF}$ is an expansion estimator in the Löwner sense. Next, we give an improved estimator shrinking $\widehat{\boldsymbol{\Sigma}}^{BS}$.

For positive constants b and c, define

$$\widehat{\boldsymbol{\Sigma}}^{SH} = \boldsymbol{H}\boldsymbol{L}\boldsymbol{\Phi}^{SH}(\boldsymbol{L})\boldsymbol{H}^\top, \quad \boldsymbol{\Phi}^{SH}(\boldsymbol{L}) = \frac{1}{\kappa}\Big(\boldsymbol{I}_\nu + \frac{b}{\operatorname{tr}\boldsymbol{L}^c}\boldsymbol{L}^c\Big)^{-1},$$

where $\boldsymbol{L}^c = \mathrm{diag}\,(\ell_1^c, \ldots, \ell_\nu^c)$. This estimator is inspired from Efron and Morris (1976) and Dey (1987) for estimating $\boldsymbol{\Sigma}^{-1}$ under certain quadratic losses. Indeed, when $n \geq p$, it corresponds to Efron and Morris (1976) for $c = 1$ and to Dey (1987) for $c = 2$. For $b > 0$, it holds that $\boldsymbol{\Phi}^{SH}(\boldsymbol{L}) \preceq \kappa^{-1}\boldsymbol{I}_\nu$, so that $\widehat{\boldsymbol{\Sigma}}^{SH} \preceq \widehat{\boldsymbol{\Sigma}}^{BS}$ in the Löwner sense. We can obtain a dominance result on the shrinkage estimator $\widehat{\boldsymbol{\Sigma}}^{SH}$ as follows.

Proposition 7.5 *For $0 < b \leq (\nu - 1)/\kappa$ and $c \geq 1$, $\widehat{\boldsymbol{\Sigma}}^{SH}$ dominates $\widehat{\boldsymbol{\Sigma}}^{BS}$ relative to the extended Stein loss* (7.3).

Proof Let $\phi_i^{SH} = \kappa^{-1}(1 + b\ell_i^c / \operatorname{tr} \boldsymbol{L}^c)^{-1}$ and $\phi_i^{SH*} = b\ell_i^c\{(1 + b)\kappa \operatorname{tr} \boldsymbol{L}^c\}^{-1}$ for $i = 1, \ldots, \nu$. Note that $\boldsymbol{\Phi}^{SH}(\boldsymbol{L}) = \mathrm{diag}\,(\phi_1^{SH}, \ldots, \phi_\nu^{SH})$ and, for $i = 1, \ldots, \nu$,

$$\begin{aligned}\phi_i^{SH} &= \kappa^{-1} - \frac{b\ell_i^c}{\kappa \operatorname{tr} \boldsymbol{L}^c}\left(1 + \frac{b\ell_i^c}{\operatorname{tr} \boldsymbol{L}^c}\right)^{-1} \\ &\leq \kappa^{-1} - \frac{b\ell_i^c}{\kappa \operatorname{tr} \boldsymbol{L}^c}(1 + b)^{-1} = \kappa^{-1} - \phi_i^{SH*}.\end{aligned}$$

Thus,

$$E[\operatorname{tr}[\mathrm{Ch}(\boldsymbol{\Sigma}^{-1}\widehat{\boldsymbol{\Sigma}}^{SH})]] \leq E[\operatorname{tr} \boldsymbol{\Sigma}^{-1}\widehat{\boldsymbol{\Sigma}}^{BS}] - E\left[\operatorname{tr} \boldsymbol{\Sigma}^{-1}\boldsymbol{H}\boldsymbol{L}\boldsymbol{\Phi}^{SH*}\boldsymbol{H}^\top\right],$$

where $\boldsymbol{\Phi}^{SH*} = \mathrm{diag}\,(\phi_1^{SH*}, \ldots, \phi_\nu^{SH*})$. It follows that

$$\begin{aligned}\log|\mathrm{Ch}(\boldsymbol{\Sigma}^{-1}\widehat{\boldsymbol{\Sigma}}^{SH})| &= \log|\mathrm{Ch}(\boldsymbol{\Sigma}^{-1}\widehat{\boldsymbol{\Sigma}}^{BS})| - \log\left|\boldsymbol{I}_\nu + \frac{b}{\operatorname{tr} \boldsymbol{L}^c}\boldsymbol{L}^c\right| \\ &\geq \log|\mathrm{Ch}(\boldsymbol{\Sigma}^{-1}\widehat{\boldsymbol{\Sigma}}^{BS})| - \operatorname{tr}\left(\frac{b}{\operatorname{tr} \boldsymbol{L}^c}\boldsymbol{L}^c\right) = \log|\mathrm{Ch}(\boldsymbol{\Sigma}^{-1}\widehat{\boldsymbol{\Sigma}}^{BS})| - b,\end{aligned}$$

so that

$$R_{ES}(\widehat{\boldsymbol{\Sigma}}^{SH}, \boldsymbol{\Sigma}) - R_{ES}(\widehat{\boldsymbol{\Sigma}}^{BS}, \boldsymbol{\Sigma}) \leq -E\left[\operatorname{tr} \boldsymbol{\Sigma}^{-1}\boldsymbol{H}\boldsymbol{L}\boldsymbol{\Phi}^{SH*}\boldsymbol{H}^\top\right] + b. \tag{7.20}$$

Using the identity (7.17) gives

$$\begin{aligned}&E\left[\operatorname{tr} \boldsymbol{\Sigma}^{-1}\boldsymbol{H}\boldsymbol{L}\boldsymbol{\Phi}^{SH*}\boldsymbol{H}^\top\right] \\ &= E\left[\sum_{i=1}^{\nu}\left\{(|n - p| + 1)\phi_i^{SH*} + 2\ell_i\frac{\partial\phi_i^{SH*}}{\partial\ell_i} + 2\sum_{j>i}^{\nu}\frac{\ell_i\phi_i^{SH*} - \ell_j\phi_j^{SH*}}{\ell_i - \ell_j}\right\}\right].\end{aligned} \tag{7.21}$$

For $b > 0$ and $c \geq 1$,

$$\sum_{i=1}^{\nu}\ell_i\frac{\partial\phi_i^{SH*}}{\partial\ell_i} = \frac{bc}{(1 + b)\kappa}\left(1 - \frac{\operatorname{tr} \boldsymbol{L}^{2c}}{(\operatorname{tr} \boldsymbol{L}^c)^2}\right) \geq 0. \tag{7.22}$$

Since, for $1 \le i < j \le \nu$ and $c \ge 1$,

$$\frac{\ell_i^{c+1} - \ell_j^{c+1}}{\ell_i - \ell_j} \ge \ell_i^c + \ell_j^c,$$

and $\sum_{i=1}^{\nu} \sum_{j>i}^{\nu} (\ell_i^c + \ell_j^c) = (\nu - 1) \operatorname{tr} \boldsymbol{L}^c$, we obtain

$$\sum_{i=1}^{\nu} \sum_{j>i}^{\nu} \frac{\ell_i \phi_i^{SH*} - \ell_j \phi_j^{SH*}}{\ell_i - \ell_j} \ge \frac{b}{(1+b)\kappa \operatorname{tr} \boldsymbol{L}^c} \sum_{i=1}^{\nu} \sum_{j>i}^{\nu} (\ell_i^c + \ell_j^c) = \frac{(\nu-1)b}{(1+b)\kappa}. \tag{7.23}$$

Combining (7.20)–(7.23) provides

$$R_{ES}(\widehat{\boldsymbol{\Sigma}}^{SH}, \boldsymbol{\Sigma}) - R_{ES}(\widehat{\boldsymbol{\Sigma}}^{BS}, \boldsymbol{\Sigma}) \le -\frac{(n+p-1)b}{(1+b)\kappa} + b = \frac{\kappa b^2 - (\nu-1)b}{(1+b)\kappa},$$

which is not positive if $0 < b \le (\nu - 1)/\kappa$. □

7.4.3.3 Stein's Simple Estimator and Risk Minimization Method

In the nonsingular case, namely, $n \ge p$, the unbiased estimator $\widehat{\boldsymbol{\Sigma}}^{UB}$ can be expressed as $\widehat{\boldsymbol{\Sigma}}^{UB} = \boldsymbol{H}\boldsymbol{L}\boldsymbol{D}_p^{UB}\boldsymbol{H}$ with $\boldsymbol{L} = \operatorname{diag}(\ell_1, \ldots, \ell_p)$ and $\boldsymbol{D}_p^{UB} = \operatorname{diag}(n^{-1}, \ldots, n^{-1})$. Then the first and last diagonal elements of $\boldsymbol{L}\boldsymbol{D}_p^{UB}$ are, respectively, ℓ_1/n and ℓ_p/n, which are the largest and smallest eigenvalues of $\widehat{\boldsymbol{\Sigma}}^{UB}$. Let λ_1 be the largest eigenvalue of $\boldsymbol{\Sigma}$ and let $\boldsymbol{\eta}$ be the corresponding normalized eigenvector. Now,

$$\lambda_1 = \boldsymbol{\eta}^\top \boldsymbol{\Sigma} \boldsymbol{\eta} = E\left[\boldsymbol{\eta}^\top \widehat{\boldsymbol{\Sigma}}^{UB} \boldsymbol{\eta}\right] \le E\left[\max_{\boldsymbol{\xi} \in \mathbb{R}^p : \|\boldsymbol{\xi}\|=1} \boldsymbol{\xi}^\top \widehat{\boldsymbol{\Sigma}}^{UB} \boldsymbol{\xi}\right] = E[\ell_1/n].$$

Similarly, it can be shown that $E[\ell_p/n] \le \lambda_p$, where λ_p is the smallest eigenvalue of $\boldsymbol{\Sigma}$. These imply that ℓ_1/n overestimates λ_1 and ℓ_p/n underestimates λ_p, so that $\widehat{\boldsymbol{\Sigma}}^{UB}$ should probably be modified by shrinking its largest eigenvalue ℓ_1/n and expanding its smallest eigenvalue ℓ_p/n. In other words, an orthogonally invariant estimator $\widehat{\boldsymbol{\Sigma}}^{O} = \boldsymbol{H}\boldsymbol{L}\boldsymbol{\Phi}(\boldsymbol{L})\boldsymbol{H}^\top$ with $\boldsymbol{\Phi}(\boldsymbol{L}) = \operatorname{diag}(\phi_1(\boldsymbol{L}), \ldots, \phi_p(\boldsymbol{L}))$ should satisfy $\phi_1(\boldsymbol{L}) \le \cdots \le \phi_p(\boldsymbol{L})$. Moreover from the eigenvalue decomposition $\boldsymbol{S} = \boldsymbol{H}\boldsymbol{L}\boldsymbol{H}^\top$, $\boldsymbol{L}$ is defined by the diagonal matrix consisting of ordered eigenvalues $\ell_1 \ge \cdots \ge \ell_p$. Thus, for the orthogonally invariant estimators $\widehat{\boldsymbol{\Sigma}}^{O}$, it seems reasonable that the $\ell_i \phi_i(\boldsymbol{L})$'s are required to have the property $\ell_1\phi_1(\boldsymbol{L}) \ge \cdots \ge \ell_p\phi_p(\boldsymbol{L})$. As in Perron (1992), the properties $\phi_1(\boldsymbol{L}) \le \cdots \le \phi_p(\boldsymbol{L})$ and $\ell_1\phi_1(\boldsymbol{L}) \ge \cdots \ge \ell_p\phi_p(\boldsymbol{L})$ shall be called, respectively, the shrinkage and ordering properties. Sheena and Takemura (1992) called $\widehat{\boldsymbol{\Sigma}}^{O}$ order-preserving when $\widehat{\boldsymbol{\Sigma}}^{O}$ has the ordering property.

Here we will provide well known, two orthogonally invariant estimators with the shrinkage and ordering properties given by Stein. For details, see Stein (1975, 1977) and also Dey and Srinivasan (1985).

The first estimator is given by

$$\widehat{\mathbf{\Sigma}}^{ST} = \boldsymbol{H}\boldsymbol{L}\boldsymbol{D}_{\nu}^{JS}\boldsymbol{H}^{\top}, \tag{7.24}$$

where $\boldsymbol{D}_{\nu}^{JS}$ is given in (7.12). Since $d_1^{JS} \leq \cdots \leq d_{\nu}^{JS}$, $\widehat{\mathbf{\Sigma}}^{ST}$ has the shrinkage property, but lacks the ordering property. As in the following proposition, the simple estimator $\widehat{\mathbf{\Sigma}}^{ST}$ improves $\widehat{\mathbf{\Sigma}}^{JS}$.

Proposition 7.6 *$\widehat{\mathbf{\Sigma}}^{ST}$ dominates $\widehat{\mathbf{\Sigma}}^{JS}$ relative to the extended Stein loss* (7.3).

Proof This proposition can be proved in the same lines as in Dey and Srinivasan (1985, Theorem 3.1). Using (7.19), we can write the difference between the unbiased risk estimate of $\widehat{\mathbf{\Sigma}}^{ST}$ and the constant risk of $\widehat{\mathbf{\Sigma}}^{JS}$ as

$$\begin{aligned}\widehat{\Delta}(\widehat{\mathbf{\Sigma}}^{ST}) &= \widehat{R}_{ES}(\widehat{\mathbf{\Sigma}}^{ST}) - R_{ES}(\widehat{\mathbf{\Sigma}}^{JS}, \mathbf{\Sigma}) \\ &= \sum_{i=1}^{\nu}\left\{(|n-p|+1)d_i^{JS} + 2\sum_{j>i}^{\nu}\frac{d_i^{JS}\ell_i - d_j^{JS}\ell_j}{\ell_i - \ell_j}\right\} - \nu.\end{aligned}$$

It is observed that

$$\begin{aligned}\sum_{i=1}^{\nu}\sum_{j>i}^{\nu}\frac{d_i^{JS}\ell_i - d_j^{JS}\ell_j}{\ell_i - \ell_j} &= \sum_{i=1}^{\nu}\sum_{j>i}^{\nu}\frac{d_i^{JS}(\ell_i - \ell_j) + (d_i^{JS} - d_j^{JS})\ell_j}{\ell_i - \ell_j} \\ &< \sum_{i=1}^{\nu}\sum_{j>i}^{\nu} d_i^{JS} = \sum_{i=1}^{\nu}(\nu - i)d_i^{JS},\end{aligned}$$

where the inequality is verified by the facts that $\ell_1 > \cdots > \ell_{\nu}$ and that $d_1^{JS} < \cdots < d_{\nu}^{JS}$. Thus,

$$\widehat{\Delta}(\widehat{\mathbf{\Sigma}}^{ST}) < \sum_{i=1}^{\nu}(|n-p|+1+2\nu-2i)d_i^{JS} - \nu = \sum_{i=1}^{\nu}(n+p-2i+1)d_i^{JS} - \nu = 0,$$

which completes the proof. □

The other well-known estimator due to Stein (1975, 1977) is obtained from minimizing the unbiased risk estimate (7.18) subject to ϕ_i's with ignoring differential terms. The unbiased risk estimate (7.18) with ignoring differential terms can be rewritten as

$$\widehat{R}_*(\widehat{\mathbf{\Sigma}}^{O}) = \sum_{i=1}^{\nu}\left\{(|n-p|+1)\phi_i + 2\sum_{j\neq i}^{\nu}\frac{\ell_i\phi_i}{\ell_i - \ell_j} - \log\phi_i\right\} + \text{const.}$$

which is minimized by, for $i = 1, \ldots, \nu$,

$$\phi_i^{RM} = 1/\omega_i(\boldsymbol{L}), \qquad \omega_i(\boldsymbol{L}) = |n-p| + 1 + 2\ell_i \sum_{j\neq i}^{\nu} \frac{1}{\ell_i - \ell_j}.$$

The ϕ_i^{RM}'s are sometimes negative and not satisfying the ordering property $\ell_1\phi_1^{RM} \geq \cdots \geq \ell_\nu\phi_\nu^{RM}$. To modify them, Stein (1977) suggested applying the isotonic regression to ϕ_i^{RM}'s. For a detailed example of the isotonic regression, see Lin and Perlman (1985). No exact dominance result exists for the resulting modified estimator with the ordering property, but it has been much used for numerical comparison in the literature including Lin and Perlman (1985), Haff (1991), Yang and Berger (1994) and Ledoit and Wolf (2004).

7.4.3.4 The Dey-Srinivasan Estimator

Next, we introduce an improved estimator, which is based on Dey and Srinivasan (1985). Let $\boldsymbol{\Phi}^{DS}(\boldsymbol{L}) = \text{diag}\,(\phi_1^{DS}, \ldots, \phi_\nu^{DS})$ with

$$\phi_i^{DS} = d_i^{JS} - \frac{g(u)\log\ell_i}{b+u}, \qquad u = \sum_{i=1}^{\nu}(\log\ell_i)^2,$$

where b is a suitable constant and $g(u)$ is a differentiable function of u. Define

$$\widehat{\boldsymbol{\Sigma}}^{DS} = \boldsymbol{H}\boldsymbol{L}\boldsymbol{\Phi}^{DS}(\boldsymbol{L})\boldsymbol{H}^\top.$$

Of course, $\phi_1^{DS} \leq \cdots \leq \phi_\nu^{DS}$, so $\widehat{\boldsymbol{\Sigma}}^{DS}$ has the shrinkage property.

Proposition 7.7 *Suppose $\nu \geq 3$ and $b \geq 144(\nu-2)^2/\{25(n+p-1)^2\}$. If $g(u)$ is nondecreasing in u and $0 < g(u) \leq 12(\nu-2)/\{5(n+p-1)^2\}$, then $\widehat{\boldsymbol{\Sigma}}^{DS}$ dominates $\widehat{\boldsymbol{\Sigma}}^{JS}$ and $\widehat{\boldsymbol{\Sigma}}^{ST}$ relative to the extended Stein loss* (7.3).

Proof From a straightforward calculation after substituting $\phi_i = \phi_i^{DS}$ into (7.18), the unbiased risk estimate of $\widehat{\boldsymbol{\Sigma}}^{DS}$ can be expressed as

$$\widehat{R}_{ES}(\widehat{\boldsymbol{\Sigma}}^{DS}) = \widehat{R}_{ES}(\widehat{\boldsymbol{\Sigma}}^{ST}) + \widehat{\Delta}^{DS},$$

where

$$\widehat{\Delta}^{DS} = \sum_{i=1}^{\nu}\Bigg\{ -(|n-p|+1)\frac{g(u)\log\ell_i}{b+u} - 2\ell_i\frac{\partial}{\partial\ell_i}\frac{g(u)\log\ell_i}{b+u} \\ - 2\frac{g(u)}{b+u}\sum_{j>i}^{\nu}\frac{\ell_i\log\ell_i - \ell_j\log\ell_j}{\ell_i-\ell_j} - \log\left(1 - \frac{g(u)\log\ell_i}{d_i^{JS}(b+u)}\right)\Bigg\}.$$

If $\widehat{\Delta}^{DS} \leq 0$ then the proposition is verified.

Note that

$$\sum_{j>i}^{\nu} \frac{\ell_i \log \ell_i - \ell_j \log \ell_j}{\ell_i - \ell_j} = (\nu - i) \log \ell_i + \sum_{j>i}^{\nu} \frac{\log \ell_i - \log \ell_j}{\ell_i - \ell_j} \ell_j \geq (\nu - i) \log \ell_i$$

because $\ell_1 \geq \cdots \geq \ell_\nu$. Further noting that

$$\ell_i \frac{\partial}{\partial \ell_i} \frac{g(u) \log \ell_i}{b+u} = \frac{g(u)}{b+u} + 2\frac{g'(u)(\log \ell_i)^2}{b+u} - 2\frac{g(u)(\log \ell_i)^2}{(b+u)^2},$$

we obtain

$$\begin{aligned} \widehat{\Delta}^{DS} \leq \sum_{i=1}^{\nu} \Bigg\{ & -\frac{g(u) \log \ell_i}{d_i^{JS}(b+u)} - 2\frac{g(u)}{b+u} - 4\frac{g'(u)(\log \ell_i)^2}{b+u} \\ & + 4\frac{g(u)(\log \ell_i)^2}{(b+u)^2} - \log\left(1 - \frac{g(u)\log \ell_i}{d_i^{JS}(b+u)}\right)\Bigg\}. \end{aligned} \tag{7.25}$$

It follows that $|x|/(b+x^2) \leq \{2\sqrt{b}\}^{-1}$ for $b > 0$, implying that for each i

$$\frac{|\log \ell_i|}{b+u} < \frac{|\log \ell_i|}{b + (\log \ell_i)^2} \leq \frac{1}{2\sqrt{b}}.$$

Combining this inequality and the given conditions on b and $g(u)$ gives

$$\frac{g(u)|\log \ell_i|}{d_i^{JS}(b+u)} \leq (n+p-1)\frac{g(u)|\log \ell_i|}{b+u} < \frac{1}{2\sqrt{b}} \times \frac{12(\nu-2)}{5(n+p-1)} < \frac{1}{2}.$$

Since

$$\log(1+x) \geq x - \frac{5}{6}x^2$$

for $|x| \leq 1/2$ (see Dey and Srinivasan 1985, Lemma 2.2), using the given condition on $g(u)$ yields

$$\begin{aligned} \log\left(1 - \frac{g(u)\log \ell_i}{d_i^{JS}(b+u)}\right) &\geq -\frac{g(u)\log \ell_i}{d_i^{JS}(b+u)} - \frac{5}{6}\left\{\frac{g(u)\log \ell_i}{d_i^{JS}(b+u)}\right\}^2 \\ &> -\frac{g(u)\log \ell_i}{d_i^{JS}(b+u)} - 2(\nu-2)\frac{g(u)(\log \ell_i)^2}{(b+u)^2}. \end{aligned} \tag{7.26}$$

Combining (7.25) and (7.26) gives

$$\widehat{\Delta}^{DS} < \sum_{i=1}^{\nu}\left\{-2\frac{g(u)}{b+u} - 4\frac{g'(u)(\log \ell_i)^2}{b+u} + 2\nu\frac{g(u)(\log \ell_i)^2}{(b+u)^2}\right\}$$

$$= -2\nu\frac{g(u)}{b+u} - 4\frac{ug'(u)}{b+u} + 2\nu\frac{ug(u)}{(b+u)^2} < -4\frac{ug'(u)}{b+u} \le 0,$$

which completes the proof. □

7.4.3.5 Sheena and Takemura's Methods for Improving Non-order-preserving Estimators

Let $\boldsymbol{\varphi} = (\varphi_1, \ldots, \varphi_\nu)$ and $\operatorname{diag}(\boldsymbol{\varphi}) = \operatorname{diag}(\varphi_1, \ldots, \varphi_\nu)$, where $\varphi_i = \ell_i \phi_i(\boldsymbol{L})$ for $i = 1, \ldots, \nu$. Here as in Sheena and Takemura (1992), we call $\widehat{\boldsymbol{\Sigma}}^{O} = \boldsymbol{H} \operatorname{diag}(\boldsymbol{\varphi})\boldsymbol{H}^\top$ order-preserving if $\widehat{\boldsymbol{\Sigma}}^{O}$ has the ordering property $\varphi_1 \ge \cdots \ge \varphi_\nu$. Note that $\widehat{\boldsymbol{\Sigma}}^{ST}$ and $\widehat{\boldsymbol{\Sigma}}^{DS}$ are not always order-preserving since $\ell_1 \ge \cdots \ge \ell_\nu$, $d_1^{JS} \le \cdots \le d_\nu^{JS}$ and $\phi_1^{DS} \le \cdots \le \phi_\nu^{DS}$. Sheena and Takemura (1992) give two methods of improving such a non-order-preserving estimator in the nonsingular case. Now, the methods are unifiedly treated for the nonsingular and singular cases:

(i) For $i = 1, \ldots, \nu$, let $\varphi_{(i)}$ be the i-th largest element in $\boldsymbol{\varphi} = (\varphi_1, \ldots, \varphi_\nu)$. Define $\widehat{\boldsymbol{\Sigma}}^{OS} = \boldsymbol{H} \operatorname{diag}(\boldsymbol{\varphi}^{OS})\boldsymbol{H}^\top$ with $\boldsymbol{\varphi}^{OS} = (\varphi_{(1)}, \ldots, \varphi_{(\nu)})$.
(ii) Denote by $(\varphi_1^{IR}, \ldots, \varphi_\nu^{IR})$ the isotonic regression of $(\varphi_1, \ldots, \varphi_\nu)$, satisfying

$$\min_{c_1 \ge \cdots \ge c_\nu} \sum_{i=1}^{\nu}(c_i - \varphi_i)^2 = \sum_{i=1}^{\nu}(\varphi_i^{IR} - \varphi_i)^2.$$

Define $\widehat{\boldsymbol{\Sigma}}^{IR} = \boldsymbol{H} \operatorname{diag}(\boldsymbol{\varphi}^{IR})\boldsymbol{H}^\top$ with $\boldsymbol{\varphi}^{IR} = (\varphi_1^{IR}, \ldots, \varphi_\nu^{IR})$.

The φ_i^{IR}'s are given by

$$\varphi_i^{IR} = \min_{s \le i} \max_{t \ge i} \frac{\sum_{r=s}^{t} \varphi_r}{t - s + 1},$$

so that $\sum_{i=1}^{\nu} g(\varphi_i^{IR}) \le \sum_{i=1}^{\nu} g(\varphi_i)$ for any convex function g. For computation algorithm and mathematical properties of the isotonic regression, see Robertson et al. (1988, Chap. 1).

We first show the following theorem.

Theorem 7.2 *Let $\widehat{\boldsymbol{\Sigma}}(\boldsymbol{\varphi}^*) = \boldsymbol{H} \operatorname{diag}(\boldsymbol{\varphi}^*)\boldsymbol{H}^\top$ be an orthogonally invariant estimator of $\boldsymbol{\Sigma}$, where $\boldsymbol{\varphi}^* = (\varphi_1^*, \ldots, \varphi_\nu^*)$ and the φ_i^*'s are functions of $\boldsymbol{L}$. Assume that*

$$\sum_{i=1}^{j} \varphi_i^* \ge \sum_{i=1}^{j} \varphi_i \quad \text{for } 1 \le j \le \nu - 1, \quad \text{and} \quad \sum_{i=1}^{\nu} \varphi_i^* = \sum_{i=1}^{\nu} \varphi_i.$$

If $\Pr(\boldsymbol{\varphi}^* = \boldsymbol{\varphi}) \neq 1$ *and* $\sum_{i=1}^{\nu} \log \varphi_i^* \geq \sum_{i=1}^{\nu} \log \varphi_i$, *then* $\widehat{\boldsymbol{\Sigma}}(\boldsymbol{\varphi}^*)$ *dominates* $\widehat{\boldsymbol{\Sigma}}(\boldsymbol{\varphi})$ *relative to the extended Stein loss* (7.3).

Proof Since $|\mathrm{Ch}(\boldsymbol{\Sigma}^{-1}\boldsymbol{H}\,\mathrm{diag}\,(\boldsymbol{\varphi}^*)\boldsymbol{H}^\top)| = |\boldsymbol{H}^\top\boldsymbol{\Sigma}^{-1}\boldsymbol{H}|\prod_{i=1}^{\nu}\varphi_i^*$, we obtain

$$\begin{aligned}\log|\mathrm{Ch}(\boldsymbol{\Sigma}^{-1}\boldsymbol{H}\,\mathrm{diag}\,(\boldsymbol{\varphi}^*)\boldsymbol{H}^\top)| &= \log|\boldsymbol{H}^\top\boldsymbol{\Sigma}^{-1}\boldsymbol{H}| + \sum_{i=1}^{\nu}\log\varphi_i^* \\ &\geq \log|\boldsymbol{H}^\top\boldsymbol{\Sigma}^{-1}\boldsymbol{H}| + \sum_{i=1}^{\nu}\log\varphi_i \\ &= \log|\mathrm{Ch}(\boldsymbol{\Sigma}^{-1}\boldsymbol{H}\,\mathrm{diag}\,(\boldsymbol{\varphi})\boldsymbol{H}^\top)|,\end{aligned}$$

so that

$$R_{ES}(\widehat{\boldsymbol{\Sigma}}(\boldsymbol{\varphi}^*), \boldsymbol{\Sigma}) - R_{ES}(\widehat{\boldsymbol{\Sigma}}(\boldsymbol{\varphi}), \boldsymbol{\Sigma}) \leq E[\mathrm{tr}\,\boldsymbol{\Sigma}^{-1}\boldsymbol{H}\{\mathrm{diag}\,(\boldsymbol{\varphi}^*) - \mathrm{diag}\,(\boldsymbol{\varphi})\}\boldsymbol{H}^\top].$$

For $i = 1, \ldots, \nu$, let $a_i = \{\boldsymbol{H}^\top\boldsymbol{\Sigma}^{-1}\boldsymbol{H}\}_{ii}$. From (3.3),

$$\begin{aligned}&E[\mathrm{tr}\,\boldsymbol{\Sigma}^{-1}\boldsymbol{H}\{\mathrm{diag}\,(\boldsymbol{\varphi}^*) - \mathrm{diag}\,(\boldsymbol{\varphi})\}\boldsymbol{H}^\top] \\ &= E\left[\sum_{i=1}^{\nu}(\varphi_i^* - \varphi_i)a_i\right] \\ &= c\int_{\mathbb{D}_\nu^{(\geq 0)}}\sum_{i=1}^{\nu}(\varphi_i^* - \varphi_i)E^*(a_i|\boldsymbol{L})|\boldsymbol{L}|^{(|n-p|-1)/2}\left(\prod_{1\leq i<j\leq\nu}(\ell_1 - \ell_j)\right)(\mathrm{d}\boldsymbol{L}),\end{aligned}$$

where c is a constant and

$$E^*(a_i|\boldsymbol{L}) = \int_{\mathbb{V}_{p,\nu}} a_i \exp\left(-\frac{1}{2}\sum_{k=1}^{\nu}a_k\ell_k\right)(\boldsymbol{H}^\top\mathrm{d}\boldsymbol{H}).$$

Note that

$$\begin{aligned}&\sum_{i=1}^{\nu}(\varphi_i^* - \varphi_i)E^*(a_i|\boldsymbol{L}) \\ &= (\varphi_1^* - \varphi_1)\{E^*(a_1|\boldsymbol{L}) - E^*(a_2|\boldsymbol{L})\} + (\varphi_1^* + \varphi_2^* - \varphi_1 - \varphi_2)\{E^*(a_2|\boldsymbol{L}) - E^*(a_3|\boldsymbol{L})\} \\ &\quad + \cdots + (\varphi_1^* + \cdots + \varphi_{\nu-1}^* - \varphi_1 - \cdots - \varphi_{\nu-1})\{E^*(a_{\nu-1}|\boldsymbol{L}) - E^*(a_\nu|\boldsymbol{L})\}.\end{aligned}$$

Hence, if

$$\Delta_i(\boldsymbol{L}) \equiv E^*(a_i|\boldsymbol{L}) - E^*(a_{i+1}|\boldsymbol{L}) \leq 0$$

for $i = 1, \ldots, \nu - 1$ then $R_{ES}(\widehat{\boldsymbol{\Sigma}}(\boldsymbol{\varphi}^*), \boldsymbol{\Sigma}) \leq R_{ES}(\widehat{\boldsymbol{\Sigma}}(\boldsymbol{\varphi}), \boldsymbol{\Sigma})$.

Since $(\boldsymbol{H}^\top\mathrm{d}\boldsymbol{H})$ is invariant under any orthogonal transformation, it is invariant under permutation of columns of $\boldsymbol{H}$. Exchanging the i-th and $(i+1)$-th columns of

$\boldsymbol{H}$ gives

$$\Delta_i(\boldsymbol{L}) = \int_{\mathbb{V}_{p,\nu}} (a_{i+1} - a_i) \exp\Big(-\frac{1}{2} a_i \ell_{i+1} - \frac{1}{2} a_{i+1} \ell_i - \frac{1}{2} \sum_{k \neq i, i+1}^{\nu} a_k \ell_k \Big) (\boldsymbol{H}^\top \mathrm{d}\boldsymbol{H}),$$

so that

$$\begin{aligned} 2\Delta_i(\boldsymbol{L}) &= \int_{\mathbb{V}_{p,\nu}} (a_i - a_{i+1}) \exp\Big(-\frac{1}{2} \sum_{k=1}^{\nu} a_k \ell_k \Big) (\boldsymbol{H}^\top \mathrm{d}\boldsymbol{H}) \\ &\quad + \int_{\mathbb{V}_{p,\nu}} (a_{i+1} - a_i) \exp\Big(-\frac{1}{2} a_i \ell_{i+1} - \frac{1}{2} a_{i+1} \ell_i - \frac{1}{2} \sum_{k \neq i, i+1}^{\nu} a_k \ell_k \Big) (\boldsymbol{H}^\top \mathrm{d}\boldsymbol{H}) \\ &= \int_{\mathbb{V}_{p,\nu}} (a_i - a_{i+1}) \Big\{ 1 - \exp\Big(\frac{1}{2} (a_i - a_{i+1})(\ell_i - \ell_{i+1}) \Big) \Big\} \\ &\qquad \times \exp\Big(-\frac{1}{2} \sum_{k=1}^{\nu} a_k \ell_k \Big) (\boldsymbol{H}^\top \mathrm{d}\boldsymbol{H}). \end{aligned}$$

For both when $a_i - a_{i+1} \geq 0$ and when $a_i - a_{i+1} < 0$, we can verify $\Delta_i(\boldsymbol{L}) \leq 0$. Thus the proof is complete. □

It is easy to check that both estimators $\widehat{\boldsymbol{\Sigma}}^{OS}$ and $\widehat{\boldsymbol{\Sigma}}^{IR}$ satisfy conditions of Theorem 7.2. Hence we obtain the following proposition.

Proposition 7.8 *$\widehat{\boldsymbol{\Sigma}}^{OS}$ and $\widehat{\boldsymbol{\Sigma}}^{IR}$ are better than $\widehat{\boldsymbol{\Sigma}}^{O}$ relative to the extended Stein loss* (7.3).

7.4.3.6 The Perron Estimator

Consider the case of $n \geq p$. For every $\boldsymbol{O} \in \mathbb{O}_p$, let $\boldsymbol{T}_O \boldsymbol{T}_O^\top$ be the Cholesky decomposition of $\boldsymbol{O}^\top \boldsymbol{S} \boldsymbol{O}$, where $\boldsymbol{T}_O \in \mathbb{L}_p^{(+)}$. Using the James-Stein estimator $\widehat{\boldsymbol{\Sigma}}^{JS} = \widehat{\boldsymbol{\Sigma}}^{JS}(\boldsymbol{S})$, we define an estimator of $\boldsymbol{\Sigma}$ as

$$\widehat{\boldsymbol{\Sigma}}^{E} = E[\boldsymbol{O} \widehat{\boldsymbol{\Sigma}}^{JS}(\boldsymbol{O}^\top \boldsymbol{S} \boldsymbol{O}) \boldsymbol{O}^\top | \boldsymbol{S}] = E[\boldsymbol{O} \boldsymbol{T}_O \boldsymbol{D}_p^{JS} \boldsymbol{T}_O^\top \boldsymbol{O}^\top | \boldsymbol{S}],$$

where $E[\cdot|\boldsymbol{S}]$ stands for conditional expectation with respect to the uniform distribution on $\mathbb{O}_p$ given $\boldsymbol{S}$. Eaton (1970) suggested that $\widehat{\boldsymbol{\Sigma}}^{E}$ is an orthogonally invariant estimator improving $\widehat{\boldsymbol{\Sigma}}^{JS}$ relative to the ordinary Stein loss (7.2). Denote $\widehat{\boldsymbol{\Sigma}}^{E} = \boldsymbol{H} \boldsymbol{L} \boldsymbol{\Phi}^{E}(\boldsymbol{L}) \boldsymbol{H}^\top$ with $\boldsymbol{\Phi}^{E}(\boldsymbol{L}) = \mathrm{diag}\,(\phi_1^E, \ldots, \phi_p^E)$. The computation of $\boldsymbol{\Phi}^{E}(\boldsymbol{L})$ was done by Sharma and Krishnamoorthy (1983) for $p = 2$ and by Takemura (1984) for $p = 3$. Takemura (1984) also provided a detailed discussion on $\widehat{\boldsymbol{\Sigma}}^{E}$ and showed that, for $i = 1, \ldots, p$, ϕ_i^E can be expressed by

$$\phi_i^E = \sum_{j=1}^{p} w_{ij}(\boldsymbol{L}) d_j^{JS},$$

where $\boldsymbol{W}(\boldsymbol{L}) = (w_{ij}(\boldsymbol{L}))$ is a doubly stochastic matrix. A closed form of $\boldsymbol{W}(\boldsymbol{L})$ is hard to clarify. Perron (1992) proposed an approximation method for $\boldsymbol{W}(\boldsymbol{L})$ and established a dominance result of the resulting estimator. Here, we give a unified Perron (1992) type estimator for the $n \geq p$ and the $p > n$ cases.

For $i, j \in \{1, \ldots, \nu\}$, let

$$w_{ij}^{PR}(\boldsymbol{L}) = \frac{\operatorname{tr}_{j-1}(\boldsymbol{L}_i)}{\operatorname{tr}_{j-1}(\boldsymbol{L})} - \frac{\operatorname{tr}_j(\boldsymbol{L}_i)}{\operatorname{tr}_j(\boldsymbol{L})},$$

where $\boldsymbol{L}_i = \operatorname{diag}(\ell_1, \ldots, \ell_{i-1}, 0, \ell_{i+1}, \ldots, \ell_\nu)$ and

$$\operatorname{tr}_j(\boldsymbol{L}) = \begin{cases} 1, & \text{if } j = 0, \\ \sum_{1 \leq i_1 < \cdots < i_j \leq \nu} \prod_{k=1}^{j} \ell_{i_k}, & \text{if } j \in \{1, \ldots, \nu\}, \\ 0, & \text{otherwise.} \end{cases}$$

Let $\phi_i^{PR} = \sum_{j=1}^{\nu} w_{ij}^{PR}(\boldsymbol{L}) d_j^{JS}$ for $i = 1, \ldots, \nu$ and let $\boldsymbol{\Phi}^{PR}(\boldsymbol{L}) = \operatorname{diag}(\phi_1^{PR}, \ldots, \phi_\nu^{PR})$. The Perron (1992) type estimator is defined by

$$\widehat{\boldsymbol{\Sigma}}^{PR} = \boldsymbol{H}\boldsymbol{L}\boldsymbol{\Phi}^{PR}(\boldsymbol{L})\boldsymbol{H}^\top.$$

Then we obtain the following proposition.

Proposition 7.9 *The Perron type estimator* $\widehat{\boldsymbol{\Sigma}}^{PR}$ *is better than* $\widehat{\boldsymbol{\Sigma}}^{JS}$ *relative to the extended Stein loss* (7.3).

The proof of Proposition 7.9 is omitted since it can be done along the same lines as in Perron (1992). A noteworthy fact is that $\widehat{\boldsymbol{\Sigma}}^{PR}$ has the ordering and shrinkage properties

$$\ell_1 \phi_1^{PR}(\boldsymbol{L}) \geq \cdots \geq \ell_\nu \phi_\nu^{PR}(\boldsymbol{L}), \quad \phi_1^{PR}(\boldsymbol{L}) \leq \cdots \leq \phi_\nu^{PR}(\boldsymbol{L}),$$

which can be shown in the same arguments as in Perron (1992). Hence $\widehat{\boldsymbol{\Sigma}}^{PR}$ is order-preserving as well.

7.5 Improvement Using Information on Mean Statistic

Kubokawa and Tsai (2006) suggested a truncation method for improving the existing estimators of $\boldsymbol{\Sigma}$ based on both $\boldsymbol{Y}$ and $\boldsymbol{X}$ in (7.1) with $n \geq p$. The truncation method was generalized by Tsukuma and Kubokawa (2016) for any possible ordering among m, n and p. This section will introduce the generalized truncation method.

7.5.1 A Class of Estimators and Its Risk Function

This section uses the same notation as in Sect. 6.3. Recall that $\nu = n \wedge p$, $\tau = m \wedge n \wedge p$ and $\boldsymbol{X}\boldsymbol{H}\boldsymbol{L}^{-1/2} = \boldsymbol{R}\boldsymbol{F}^{1/2}\boldsymbol{V}^\top$, where $\boldsymbol{R} \in \mathbb{V}_{m,\tau}$, $\boldsymbol{V} \in \mathbb{V}_{\nu,\tau}$ and $\boldsymbol{F}^{1/2} = \mathrm{diag}\,(\sqrt{f_1}, \ldots, \sqrt{f_\tau}) \in \mathbb{D}_\tau^{(\geq 0)}$. As seen in Lemma 6.3, $\boldsymbol{Q}^- = \boldsymbol{V}^\top\boldsymbol{L}^{1/2}\boldsymbol{H}^\top$ is the generalized inverse of $\boldsymbol{Q} = \boldsymbol{H}\boldsymbol{L}^{-1/2}\boldsymbol{V}$.

Let $c_0 = \kappa^{-1} = (n \vee p)^{-1}$. A class of estimators treated in this section is of the form

$$\widehat{\boldsymbol{\Sigma}}(\boldsymbol{\Psi}) = \widehat{\boldsymbol{\Sigma}}^{BS} + c_0(\boldsymbol{Q}^-)^\top\boldsymbol{\Psi}(\boldsymbol{F})\boldsymbol{Q}^- = c_0\{\boldsymbol{S} + (\boldsymbol{Q}^-)^\top\boldsymbol{\Psi}(\boldsymbol{F})\boldsymbol{Q}^-\}, \tag{7.27}$$

where $\boldsymbol{\Psi}(\boldsymbol{F}) \in \mathbb{D}_\tau$ satisfies $\boldsymbol{\Psi}(\boldsymbol{F}) + \boldsymbol{I}_\tau$ is positive definite and the diagonal elements of $\boldsymbol{\Psi}(\boldsymbol{F})$ are absolutely continuous functions of $\boldsymbol{F}$. The class (7.27) can be rewritten by

$$\widehat{\boldsymbol{\Sigma}}(\boldsymbol{\Psi}) = \widehat{\boldsymbol{\Sigma}}^{BS} + c_0\boldsymbol{S}\boldsymbol{S}^+\boldsymbol{X}^\top\boldsymbol{R}\boldsymbol{F}^{-1}\boldsymbol{\Psi}(\boldsymbol{F})\boldsymbol{R}^\top\boldsymbol{X}\boldsymbol{S}\boldsymbol{S}^+$$

because $\boldsymbol{Q}^- = \boldsymbol{F}^{-1/2}\boldsymbol{R}^\top\boldsymbol{X}\boldsymbol{S}\boldsymbol{S}^+$ from (6.14). Also, the definition of $\boldsymbol{Q}^-$ implies that

$$\widehat{\boldsymbol{\Sigma}}(\boldsymbol{\Psi}) = c_0\boldsymbol{H}\boldsymbol{L}^{1/2}(\boldsymbol{I}_\nu + \boldsymbol{V}\boldsymbol{\Psi}(\boldsymbol{F})\boldsymbol{V}^\top)\boldsymbol{L}^{1/2}\boldsymbol{H}^\top.$$

When $\boldsymbol{\Psi}(\boldsymbol{F}) + \boldsymbol{I}_\tau$ is positive definite, $\boldsymbol{I}_\nu + \boldsymbol{V}\boldsymbol{\Psi}(\boldsymbol{F})\boldsymbol{V}^\top$ is positive definite and thus both $\widehat{\boldsymbol{\Sigma}}(\boldsymbol{\Psi})$ and $\boldsymbol{\Sigma}^{-1}\widehat{\boldsymbol{\Sigma}}(\boldsymbol{\Psi})$ are of rank ν with probability one. Here, we will give a useful risk expression for $\widehat{\boldsymbol{\Sigma}}(\boldsymbol{\Psi})$ in the following theorem.

Theorem 7.3 *Let $\tau = m \wedge n \wedge p$ and $\boldsymbol{\Psi} = \boldsymbol{\Psi}(\boldsymbol{F}) = \mathrm{diag}\,(\psi_1, \ldots, \psi_\tau)$. For any order among m, n and p, the risk function of $\widehat{\boldsymbol{\Sigma}}(\boldsymbol{\Psi})$ in* (7.27) *relative to the extended Stein loss* (7.3) *is expressed as*

$$\begin{aligned} R_{ES}(\widehat{\boldsymbol{\Sigma}}(\boldsymbol{\Psi}), \boldsymbol{\Sigma}) =& R_{ES}(\widehat{\boldsymbol{\Sigma}}^{BS}, \boldsymbol{\Sigma}) \\ &+ c_0 E\Bigg[\sum_{i=1}^{\tau}\alpha_i\psi_i - 2g_1(\boldsymbol{\Psi}) - 2g_2(\boldsymbol{\Psi}) - c_0^{-1}\log|\boldsymbol{I}_\tau + \boldsymbol{\Psi}|\Bigg], \end{aligned} \tag{7.28}$$

where $\alpha_i = |n - p| + 2i - 1$ for $i = 1, \ldots, \tau$ and

$$g_1(\boldsymbol{\Psi}) = \sum_{i=1}^{\tau} f_i\frac{\partial\psi_i}{\partial f_i}, \qquad g_2(\boldsymbol{\Psi}) = \sum_{i=1}^{\tau}\sum_{j>i}^{\tau}\frac{\psi_i - \psi_j}{f_i - f_j}f_j.$$

Proof Both $\boldsymbol{L}^{1/2}\boldsymbol{H}^\top\boldsymbol{\Sigma}^{-1}\boldsymbol{H}\boldsymbol{L}^{1/2}$ and $\boldsymbol{I}_\nu + \boldsymbol{V}\boldsymbol{\Psi}\boldsymbol{V}^\top$ are of rank ν, so that

$$\begin{aligned} |\mathrm{Ch}(\boldsymbol{\Sigma}^{-1}\widehat{\boldsymbol{\Sigma}}(\boldsymbol{\Psi}))| &= |\mathrm{Ch}(c_0\boldsymbol{L}^{1/2}\boldsymbol{H}^\top\boldsymbol{\Sigma}^{-1}\boldsymbol{H}\boldsymbol{L}^{1/2}(\boldsymbol{I}_\nu + \boldsymbol{V}\boldsymbol{\Psi}\boldsymbol{V}^\top))| \\ &= |c_0\boldsymbol{L}^{1/2}\boldsymbol{H}^\top\boldsymbol{\Sigma}^{-1}\boldsymbol{H}\boldsymbol{L}^{1/2}(\boldsymbol{I}_\nu + \boldsymbol{V}\boldsymbol{\Psi}\boldsymbol{V}^\top)| \\ &= |c_0\boldsymbol{L}^{1/2}\boldsymbol{H}^\top\boldsymbol{\Sigma}^{-1}\boldsymbol{H}\boldsymbol{L}^{1/2}| \times |\boldsymbol{I}_\nu + \boldsymbol{V}\boldsymbol{\Psi}\boldsymbol{V}^\top| \\ &= |\mathrm{Ch}(\boldsymbol{\Sigma}^{-1}\widehat{\boldsymbol{\Sigma}}^{BS})| \times |\boldsymbol{I}_\tau + \boldsymbol{\Psi}|. \end{aligned}$$

Since $\mathrm{tr}\,[\mathrm{Ch}(\boldsymbol{\Sigma}^{-1}\widehat{\boldsymbol{\Sigma}}^{BS})] = \mathrm{tr}\,\boldsymbol{\Sigma}^{-1}\widehat{\boldsymbol{\Sigma}}^{BS}$ and $\mathrm{tr}\,[\mathrm{Ch}(\boldsymbol{\Sigma}^{-1}\widehat{\boldsymbol{\Sigma}}(\boldsymbol{\Psi}))] = \mathrm{tr}\,\boldsymbol{\Sigma}^{-1}\widehat{\boldsymbol{\Sigma}}(\boldsymbol{\Psi})$, the risk of $\widehat{\boldsymbol{\Sigma}}(\boldsymbol{\Psi})$ with respect to the extended Stein loss (7.3) is written as

$$\begin{aligned}
R_{ES}(\widehat{\boldsymbol{\Sigma}}(\boldsymbol{\Psi}), \boldsymbol{\Sigma}) &= E[L_{ES}(\widehat{\boldsymbol{\Sigma}}(\boldsymbol{\Psi}), \boldsymbol{\Sigma})] \\
&= E[\mathrm{tr}\,[\mathrm{Ch}(\boldsymbol{\Sigma}^{-1}\widehat{\boldsymbol{\Sigma}}(\boldsymbol{\Psi}))] - \log|\mathrm{Ch}(\boldsymbol{\Sigma}^{-1}\widehat{\boldsymbol{\Sigma}}(\boldsymbol{\Psi}))| - \nu] \\
&= E[\mathrm{tr}\,\boldsymbol{\Sigma}^{-1}\widehat{\boldsymbol{\Sigma}}^{BS} - \log|\mathrm{Ch}(\boldsymbol{\Sigma}^{-1}\widehat{\boldsymbol{\Sigma}}^{BS})| - \nu] \\
&\quad + c_0 E[\mathrm{tr}\,\boldsymbol{\Sigma}^{-1}(\boldsymbol{Q}^-)^\top \boldsymbol{\Psi}\boldsymbol{Q}^- - c_0^{-1}\log|\boldsymbol{I}_\tau + \boldsymbol{\Psi}|] \\
&= R_{ES}(\widehat{\boldsymbol{\Sigma}}^{BS}, \boldsymbol{\Sigma}) + c_0 E[\mathrm{tr}\,\boldsymbol{\Sigma}^{-1}(\boldsymbol{Q}^-)^\top \boldsymbol{\Psi}\boldsymbol{Q}^- - c_0^{-1}\log|\boldsymbol{I}_\tau + \boldsymbol{\Psi}|].
\end{aligned} \tag{7.29}$$

Applying the Stein identity (5.3) and Lemma 6.7 to $E[\mathrm{tr}\,\boldsymbol{\Sigma}^{-1}(\boldsymbol{Q}^-)^\top \boldsymbol{\Psi}\boldsymbol{Q}^-]$ leads to

$$\begin{aligned}
E[\mathrm{tr}\,\boldsymbol{\Sigma}^{-1}(\boldsymbol{Q}^-)^\top \boldsymbol{\Psi}\boldsymbol{Q}^-] &= E[\mathrm{tr}\,\boldsymbol{\Sigma}^{-1}\boldsymbol{S}\boldsymbol{S}^+\boldsymbol{X}^\top \boldsymbol{R}\boldsymbol{F}^{-1}\boldsymbol{\Psi}\boldsymbol{R}^\top \boldsymbol{X}\boldsymbol{S}\boldsymbol{S}^+] \\
&= E\left[\sum_{i=1}^{\tau}\left\{a\psi_i - 2f_i\frac{\partial\psi_i}{\partial f_i} - 2\sum_{j>i}^{\tau}\frac{f_i\psi_i - f_j\psi_j}{f_i - f_j}\right\}\right],
\end{aligned}$$

where $a = n + p - 2\nu + 2\tau - 1$. It follows that

$$\sum_{i=1}^{\tau}\sum_{j>i}^{\tau}\frac{f_i\psi_i - f_j\psi_j}{f_i - f_j} = \sum_{i=1}^{\tau}\left\{(\tau - i)\psi_i + \sum_{j>i}^{\tau}\frac{\psi_i - \psi_j}{f_i - f_j}f_j\right\},$$

implying that

$$E[\mathrm{tr}\,\boldsymbol{\Sigma}^{-1}(\boldsymbol{Q}^-)^\top \boldsymbol{\Psi}\boldsymbol{Q}^-] = E\left[\sum_{i=1}^{\tau}\left\{\alpha_i\psi_i - 2f_i\frac{\partial\psi_i}{\partial f_i} - 2\sum_{j>i}^{\tau}\frac{\psi_i - \psi_j}{f_i - f_j}f_j\right\}\right]. \tag{7.30}$$

where $\alpha_i = a - 2(\tau - i) = |n - p| + 2i - 1$. Combining (7.29) and (7.30), we obtain (7.28). Thus the proof is complete. □

7.5.2 *Examples of Improved Estimators*

7.5.2.1 The Stein-Type Estimator

A Stein-type estimator similar to (7.24) is described by

$$\widehat{\boldsymbol{\Sigma}}(\boldsymbol{\Psi}^{ST}) = c_0\{\boldsymbol{S} + (\boldsymbol{Q}^-)^\top \boldsymbol{\Psi}^{ST}(\boldsymbol{F})\boldsymbol{Q}^-\}, \quad \boldsymbol{\Psi}^{ST}(\boldsymbol{F}) = \mathrm{diag}\,(\psi_1^{ST}, \dots, \psi_\tau^{ST}),$$

where for $i = 1, \dots, \tau$,

$$\psi_i^{ST} = \frac{1}{c_0\alpha_i} - 1 = \frac{\nu - 2i + 1}{|n-p| + 2i - 1}.$$

The risk function of $\widehat{\boldsymbol{\Sigma}}(\boldsymbol{\Psi}^{ST})$ under the extended Stein loss (7.3) is expressed as

$$R_{ES}(\widehat{\boldsymbol{\Sigma}}(\boldsymbol{\Psi}^{ST}), \boldsymbol{\Sigma}) = R_{ES}(\widehat{\boldsymbol{\Sigma}}^{BS}, \boldsymbol{\Sigma}) + \sum_{i=1}^{\tau}\{c_0\alpha_i\psi_i^{ST} - \log(1+\psi_i^{ST})\} - 2c_0E\big[g_2(\boldsymbol{\Psi}^{ST})\big].$$

It is observed that $\psi_i^{ST} - \psi_j^{ST} > 0$ for $j > i$, so that $g_2(\boldsymbol{\Psi}^{ST}) > 0$. Also, we see that for $i = 1, \ldots, \tau$

$$c_0\alpha_i\psi_i^{ST} - \log(1+\psi_i^{ST}) = -\{c_0\alpha_i - \log(c_0\alpha_i) - 1\} \le 0$$

because $x - \log x - 1 \ge 0$ for $x > 0$. Thus from Theorem 7.3, $\widehat{\boldsymbol{\Sigma}}(\boldsymbol{\Psi}^{ST})$ dominates $\widehat{\boldsymbol{\Sigma}}^{BS}$ for any order of m, n and p.

Further, if $\tau = \nu$, namely, $m > n \wedge p$, then $\widehat{\boldsymbol{\Sigma}}(\boldsymbol{\Psi}^{ST})$ dominates the James-Stein estimator $\widehat{\boldsymbol{\Sigma}}^{JS}$ in (7.12). In fact, since $\sum_{i=1}^{\nu}(c_0\alpha_i - 1) = 0$ and

$$\sum_{i=1}^{\nu}\log(c_0\alpha_i) = -\nu\log\kappa + \sum_{i=1}^{\nu}\log\alpha_i = -\nu\log\kappa + \sum_{i=1}^{\nu}\log(n+p-2i+1),$$

it follows that, by (7.5) and (7.13),

$$\begin{aligned} R_{ES}(\widehat{\boldsymbol{\Sigma}}(\boldsymbol{\Psi}^{ST}), \boldsymbol{\Sigma}) &< R_{ES}(\widehat{\boldsymbol{\Sigma}}^{BS}, \boldsymbol{\Sigma}) - \sum_{i=1}^{\nu}\{c_0\alpha_i - \log(c_0\alpha_i) - 1\} \\ &= \sum_{i=1}^{\nu}\log(n+p-2i+1) - r_{\kappa,\nu} = R_{ES}(\widehat{\boldsymbol{\Sigma}}^{JS}, \boldsymbol{\Sigma}). \end{aligned}$$

This shows that if $\tau = \nu$ then $\widehat{\boldsymbol{\Sigma}}(\boldsymbol{\Psi}^{ST})$ dominates $\widehat{\boldsymbol{\Sigma}}^{JS}$ relative to the extended Stein loss (7.3).

7.5.2.2 The Haff Type Estimator

As a reasonable estimator, we define the Haff (1980) type estimator as

$$\begin{aligned} &\widehat{\boldsymbol{\Sigma}}(\boldsymbol{\Psi}^{HF}) = c_0\{\boldsymbol{S} + (\boldsymbol{Q}^-)^\top\boldsymbol{\Psi}^{HF}\boldsymbol{Q}^-\}, \quad \boldsymbol{\Psi}^{HF}(\boldsymbol{F}) = \mathrm{diag}\,(\psi_1^{HF}, \ldots, \psi_\tau^{HF}), \\ &\psi_i^{HF} = \frac{a}{\mathrm{tr}\,\boldsymbol{F}}f_i \quad (i = 1, \ldots, \tau), \quad a > 0. \end{aligned}$$

Using Theorem 7.3, we can show that the Haff type estimator $\widehat{\boldsymbol{\Sigma}}(\boldsymbol{\Psi}^{HF})$ dominates $\widehat{\boldsymbol{\Sigma}}^{BS}$ if constant a satisfies the inequality $0 < a \le 2(\nu-1)/(|n-p|+1)$ for $\nu > 1$.

In fact, it is noted that

$$g_2(\boldsymbol{\Psi}^{HF}) = \sum_{i=1}^{\tau}\sum_{j>i}^{\tau}\frac{\psi_i^{HF}-\psi_j^{HF}}{f_i-f_j}f_j = \frac{a}{\operatorname{tr}\boldsymbol{F}}\sum_{i=1}^{\tau}\sum_{j>i}^{\tau}f_j = \frac{a}{\operatorname{tr}\boldsymbol{F}}\sum_{i=1}^{\tau}(i-1)f_i.$$

The difference in risk of $\widehat{\boldsymbol{\Sigma}}(\boldsymbol{\Psi}^{HF})$ and $\widehat{\boldsymbol{\Sigma}}^{BS}$ is written as

$$\begin{aligned}&R_{ES}(\widehat{\boldsymbol{\Sigma}}(\boldsymbol{\Psi}^{HF}),\boldsymbol{\Sigma}) - R_{ES}(\widehat{\boldsymbol{\Sigma}}^{BS},\boldsymbol{\Sigma})\\ &= c_0(|n-p|+1)a - 2c_0E[g_1(\boldsymbol{\Psi}^{HF})] - E\left[\sum_{i=1}^{\tau}\log(1+\psi_i^{HF})\right].\end{aligned}$$

It follows that for any $\boldsymbol{F}\in\mathbb{D}_\tau^{(\geq 0)}$

$$g_1(\boldsymbol{\Psi}^{HF}) = a\Big(1-\frac{\operatorname{tr}\boldsymbol{F}^2}{(\operatorname{tr}\boldsymbol{F})^2}\Big)\geq 0.$$

Since $\log(1+x)\geq 2x/(2+x)$ for $x\geq 0$ and $\sum_{i=1}^{\tau}\psi_i^{HF}=a$, we observe

$$\sum_{i=1}^{\tau}\log(1+\psi_i^{HF})\geq\sum_{i=1}^{\tau}\frac{2\psi_i^{HF}}{2+\psi_i^{HF}}\geq\sum_{i=1}^{\tau}\frac{2\psi_i^{HF}}{2+a}=\frac{2a}{2+a}.$$

Thus,

$$\begin{aligned}R_{ES}(\widehat{\boldsymbol{\Sigma}}(\boldsymbol{\Psi}^{HF}),\boldsymbol{\Sigma}) - R_{ES}(\widehat{\boldsymbol{\Sigma}}^{BS},\boldsymbol{\Sigma}) &\leq c_0\left\{(|n-p|+1)a - c_0^{-1}\frac{2a}{2+a}\right\}\\ &= c_0(|n-p|+1)\frac{a}{2+a}\left[a-\frac{2(\nu-1)}{|n-p|+1}\right],\end{aligned}$$

which shows the dominance result.

7.5.3 Further Improvements with a Truncation Rule

First, we provide a useful lemma which will be a key tool to show further dominance results.

Lemma 7.1 *Let $\boldsymbol{\Phi}(\boldsymbol{F})\in\mathbb{D}_\tau$ such that the diagonal elements are absolutely continuous and nonnegative functions of $\boldsymbol{F}$. Then we have*

$$E[\operatorname{tr}\boldsymbol{\Sigma}^{-1}(\boldsymbol{Q}^-)^\top(\boldsymbol{I}_\tau+\boldsymbol{F})\boldsymbol{\Phi}(\boldsymbol{F})\boldsymbol{Q}^-]\geq E[(\kappa+m)\operatorname{tr}\boldsymbol{\Phi}(\boldsymbol{F})].$$

Proof See Tsukuma and Kubokawa (2016). □

By using Lemma 7.1, we will improve on $\widehat{\boldsymbol{\Sigma}}(\boldsymbol{\Psi}^{ST})$ and $\widehat{\boldsymbol{\Sigma}}(\boldsymbol{\Psi}^{HF})$. Let $[\boldsymbol{\Psi}]^{TR} = \mathrm{diag}\,(\psi_1^{TR}(\boldsymbol{F}), \ldots, \psi_\tau^{TR}(\boldsymbol{F})) \in \mathbb{D}_\tau$ such that the i-th diagonal element is given by

$$\psi_i^{TR}(\boldsymbol{F}) = \min\left\{\psi_i(\boldsymbol{F}), \frac{1+f_i}{c_0(\kappa+m)} - 1\right\},$$

where $\boldsymbol{\Psi}(\boldsymbol{F}) = \mathrm{diag}\,(\psi_1(\boldsymbol{F}), \ldots, \psi_\tau(\boldsymbol{F}))$. Then we obtain a general dominance result for improvement on the class (7.27).

Theorem 7.4 *For any possible ordering among m, n and p, the truncated estimator* $\widehat{\boldsymbol{\Sigma}}([\boldsymbol{\Psi}]^{TR})$ *dominates* $\widehat{\boldsymbol{\Sigma}}(\boldsymbol{\Psi})$ *relative to the extended Stein loss* (7.3) *if* $\Pr([\boldsymbol{\Psi}]^{TR} \neq \boldsymbol{\Psi}) > 0$.

Proof Abbreviate $\boldsymbol{\Psi}(\boldsymbol{F})$ to $\boldsymbol{\Psi}$. The difference in risk of $\widehat{\boldsymbol{\Sigma}}(\boldsymbol{\Psi})$ and $\widehat{\boldsymbol{\Sigma}}([\boldsymbol{\Psi}]^{TR})$ can be expressed as

$$\begin{aligned}
&R_{ES}(\widehat{\boldsymbol{\Sigma}}(\boldsymbol{\Psi}), \boldsymbol{\Sigma}) - R_{ES}(\widehat{\boldsymbol{\Sigma}}([\boldsymbol{\Psi}]^{TR}), \boldsymbol{\Sigma}) \\
&= E[c_0 \,\mathrm{tr}\, \boldsymbol{\Sigma}^{-1}(\boldsymbol{Q}^-)^\top(\boldsymbol{\Psi} - [\boldsymbol{\Psi}]^{TR})\boldsymbol{Q}^- - \log|\boldsymbol{I}_\tau + \boldsymbol{\Psi}| + \log|\boldsymbol{I}_\tau + [\boldsymbol{\Psi}]^{TR}|] \\
&\geq E[c_0(\kappa+m)\,\mathrm{tr}\,(\boldsymbol{I}_\tau + \boldsymbol{F})^{-1}(\boldsymbol{\Psi} - [\boldsymbol{\Psi}]^{TR}) - \log|\boldsymbol{I}_\tau + \boldsymbol{\Psi}| + \log|\boldsymbol{I}_\tau + [\boldsymbol{\Psi}]^{TR}|],
\end{aligned}$$

where the inequality follows directly from Lemma 7.1. The last r.h.s. can be written by $E[\sum_{i=1}^{\tau} \Delta_i]$ with

$$\Delta_i = c_0(\kappa+m)\cdot\frac{\psi_i - \psi_i^{TR}}{1+f_i} - \log(1+\psi_i) + \log(1+\psi_i^{TR}).$$

When $\psi_i^{TR} = \psi_i$, we get $\Delta_i = 0$. When $\psi_i^{TR} = c_0^{-1}(1+f_i)/(\kappa+m) - 1 < \psi_i$, it is observed that

$$\Delta_i = c_0(\kappa+m)\cdot\frac{1+\psi_i}{1+f_i} - \log\left[c_0(\kappa+m)\cdot\frac{1+\psi_i}{1+f_i}\right] - 1 \geq 0,$$

which completes the proof. □

The following proposition is derived immediately from Theorem 7.4.

Proposition 7.10 *The truncated estimator* $\widehat{\boldsymbol{\Sigma}}([\boldsymbol{\Psi}^{ST}]^{TR})$ *dominates* $\widehat{\boldsymbol{\Sigma}}(\boldsymbol{\Psi}^{ST})$ *relative to the extended Stein loss* (7.3). *Also,* $\widehat{\boldsymbol{\Sigma}}([\boldsymbol{\Psi}^{HF}]^{TR})$ *dominates* $\widehat{\boldsymbol{\Sigma}}(\boldsymbol{\Psi}^{HF})$ *relative to the extended Stein loss* (7.3).

7.6 Related Topics

7.6.1 Decomposition of the Estimation Problem

When $n \geq p$, covariance estimation under the ordinary Stein loss (7.2) is closely related to simultaneous estimation of mean vectors and variances. Here we will briefly introduce the relationship and then give a simple improved procedure on $\widehat{\boldsymbol{\Sigma}}^{JS}$ via the James-Stein (1961) shrinkage estimators of multivariate normal mean vectors.

We use the same notation as in Proposition 3.10 for $n \geq p$. Recall that $\boldsymbol{T}\boldsymbol{T}^\top$ and $\boldsymbol{\Xi}\boldsymbol{\Xi}^\top$ are the Cholesky decompositions of the Wishart matrix $\boldsymbol{S}$ and the covariance matrix $\boldsymbol{\Sigma}$, respectively, where $\boldsymbol{T} = (t_{i,j}) \in \mathbb{L}_p^{(+)}$ and $\boldsymbol{\Xi} = (\xi_{i,j}) \in \mathbb{L}_p^{(+)}$. Denote $\boldsymbol{T}_{(p)} = t_{p,p}$ and $\boldsymbol{\Xi}_{(p)} = \xi_{p,p}$ and, for $i = p-1, \ldots, 1$, define $\boldsymbol{T}_{(i)}$ and $\boldsymbol{\Xi}_{(i)}$ inductively as, respectively,

$$\boldsymbol{T}_{(i)} = \begin{pmatrix} t_{i,i} & \boldsymbol{0}_{p-i}^\top \\ \boldsymbol{t}_{(i)} & \boldsymbol{T}_{(i+1)} \end{pmatrix} \in \mathbb{L}_{p-i+1}^{(+)}, \qquad \boldsymbol{\Xi}_{(i)} = \begin{pmatrix} \xi_{i,i} & \boldsymbol{0}_{p-i}^\top \\ \boldsymbol{\xi}_{(i)} & \boldsymbol{\Xi}_{(i+1)} \end{pmatrix} \in \mathbb{L}_{p-i+1}^{(+)}$$

with $\boldsymbol{t}_{(i)} = (t_{i+1,i}, \ldots, t_{p,i})^\top$ and $\boldsymbol{\xi}_{(i)} = (\xi_{i+1,i}, \ldots, \xi_{p,i})^\top$. Note that $\boldsymbol{T}_{(1)} = \boldsymbol{T}$ and $\boldsymbol{\Xi}_{(1)} = \boldsymbol{\Xi}$. By Proposition 3.10, the columns of $\boldsymbol{T}$ are mutually independent and

$$\begin{cases} t_{i,i}^2 \sim \sigma_i^2 \chi_{n-i+1}^2 & \text{for } i = 1, \ldots, p, \\ \boldsymbol{t}_{(i)} | t_{i,i} \sim \mathcal{N}_{p-i}(t_{i,i}\boldsymbol{\gamma}_{(i)}, \boldsymbol{\Sigma}_{(i+1)}) & \text{for } i = 1, \ldots, p-1, \end{cases} \tag{7.31}$$

where $\boldsymbol{\gamma}_{(i)} = \boldsymbol{\xi}_{(i)}/\xi_{i,i}$ for $i = 1, \ldots, p-1$, $\sigma_i^2 = \xi_{i,i}^2$ for $i = 1, \ldots, p$, and $\boldsymbol{\Sigma}_{(i)} = \boldsymbol{\Xi}_{(i)}\boldsymbol{\Xi}_{(i)}^\top$ for $i = 1, \ldots, p$. Recall also that for $i = 1, \ldots, p-1$

$$\boldsymbol{\Sigma}_{(i)} = \begin{pmatrix} 1 & \boldsymbol{0}_{p-i}^\top \\ \boldsymbol{\gamma}_{(i)} & \boldsymbol{I}_{p-i} \end{pmatrix} \begin{pmatrix} \sigma_i^2 & \boldsymbol{0}_{p-i}^\top \\ \boldsymbol{0}_{p-i} & \boldsymbol{\Sigma}_{(i+1)} \end{pmatrix} \begin{pmatrix} 1 & \boldsymbol{\gamma}_{(i)}^\top \\ \boldsymbol{0}_{p-i} & \boldsymbol{I}_{p-i} \end{pmatrix}. \tag{7.32}$$

Let the $\widehat{\sigma}_i^2$'s and the $\widehat{\boldsymbol{\gamma}}_{(i)}$'s be certain estimators of the σ_i^2's and the $\boldsymbol{\gamma}_{(i)}$'s, respectively. Set $\widehat{\boldsymbol{\Sigma}}_{(p)} = \widehat{\sigma}_p^2$. For $i = p-1, \ldots, 1$, we define $\widehat{\boldsymbol{\Sigma}}_{(i)}$ $(\in \mathbb{S}_{p-i+1}^{(+)})$ inductively as

$$\widehat{\boldsymbol{\Sigma}}_{(i)} = \begin{pmatrix} 1 & \boldsymbol{0}_{p-i}^\top \\ \widehat{\boldsymbol{\gamma}}_{(i)} & \boldsymbol{I}_{p-i} \end{pmatrix} \begin{pmatrix} \widehat{\sigma}_i^2 & \boldsymbol{0}_{p-i}^\top \\ \boldsymbol{0}_{p-i} & \widehat{\boldsymbol{\Sigma}}_{(i+1)} \end{pmatrix} \begin{pmatrix} 1 & \widehat{\boldsymbol{\gamma}}_{(i)}^\top \\ \boldsymbol{0}_{p-i} & \boldsymbol{I}_{p-i} \end{pmatrix}. \tag{7.33}$$

Then $\widehat{\boldsymbol{\Sigma}}^A = \widehat{\boldsymbol{\Sigma}}_{(1)}$ is an estimator of $\boldsymbol{\Sigma}$. Conversely, for any estimator $\widehat{\boldsymbol{\Sigma}}$, the LDL$^\top$ decomposition of $\widehat{\boldsymbol{\Sigma}}$ can be obtained uniquely from (7.33).

Combining (7.32) and (7.33) yields

$$\operatorname{tr} \boldsymbol{\Sigma}_{(i)}^{-1}\widehat{\boldsymbol{\Sigma}}_{(i)} = \widehat{\sigma}_i^2/\sigma_i^2 + \widehat{\sigma}_i^2(\widehat{\boldsymbol{\gamma}}_{(i)} - \boldsymbol{\gamma}_{(i)})^\top \boldsymbol{\Sigma}_{(i+1)}^{-1}(\widehat{\boldsymbol{\gamma}}_{(i)} - \boldsymbol{\gamma}_{(i)}) + \operatorname{tr} \boldsymbol{\Sigma}_{(i+1)}^{-1}\widehat{\boldsymbol{\Sigma}}_{(i+1)},$$

which is used again and again to obtain

$$\mathrm{tr}\, \boldsymbol{\Sigma}^{-1}\widehat{\boldsymbol{\Sigma}}^A = \sum_{i=1}^{p} \frac{\widehat{\sigma}_i^2}{\sigma_i^2} + \sum_{i=1}^{p-1} \widehat{\sigma}_i^2 (\widehat{\boldsymbol{\gamma}}_{(i)} - \boldsymbol{\gamma}_{(i)})^\top \boldsymbol{\Sigma}_{(i+1)}^{-1} (\widehat{\boldsymbol{\gamma}}_{(i)} - \boldsymbol{\gamma}_{(i)}).$$

Since $|\boldsymbol{\Sigma}^{-1}\boldsymbol{\Sigma}^A| = \sum_{i=1}^p \widehat{\sigma}_i^2/\sigma_i^2$, the ordinary Stein loss (7.2) of $\widehat{\boldsymbol{\Sigma}}^A$ derived from (7.33) can alternatively be written as

$$L_S(\widehat{\boldsymbol{\Sigma}}^A, \boldsymbol{\Sigma}) = \sum_{i=1}^{p} \left(\frac{\widehat{\sigma}_i^2}{\sigma_i^2} - \log \frac{\widehat{\sigma}_i^2}{\sigma_i^2} - 1 \right) + \sum_{i=1}^{p-1} \widehat{\sigma}_i^2 (\widehat{\boldsymbol{\gamma}}_{(i)} - \boldsymbol{\gamma}_{(i)})^\top \boldsymbol{\Sigma}_{(i+1)}^{-1} (\widehat{\boldsymbol{\gamma}}_{(i)} - \boldsymbol{\gamma}_{(i)}). \tag{7.34}$$

This suggests that the covariance estimation problem with the ordinary Stein loss (7.2) is considered as the problem of simultaneously estimating the σ_i^2's and the $\boldsymbol{\gamma}_{(i)}$'s under the decomposed loss (7.34) in the decomposed model (7.31).

If $\widehat{\boldsymbol{\Sigma}}^A = \widehat{\boldsymbol{\Sigma}}^{JS}$, then estimators of the σ_i^2's and the $\boldsymbol{\gamma}_{(i)}$'s can be written as, respectively,

$$\begin{cases} \widehat{\sigma}_i^{2JS} = d_i^{JS} t_{i,i}^2 & \text{for } i = 1, \ldots, p, \\ \widehat{\boldsymbol{\gamma}}_{(i)}^{JS} = \boldsymbol{t}_{(i)}/t_{i,i} & \text{for } i = 1, \ldots, p-1. \end{cases}$$

Hence the risk of $\widehat{\boldsymbol{\Sigma}}^{JS}$ is expressed by $R_S(\widehat{\boldsymbol{\Sigma}}^{JS}, \boldsymbol{\Sigma}) = E[L_S(\widehat{\boldsymbol{\Sigma}}^{JS}, \boldsymbol{\Sigma})] = R_1^{JS} + R_2^{JS}$, where

$$R_1^{JS} = E\left[\sum_{i=1}^{p} \left(\frac{\widehat{\sigma}_i^{2JS}}{\sigma_i^2} - \log \frac{\widehat{\sigma}_i^{2JS}}{\sigma_i^2} - 1 \right) \right],$$

$$R_2^{JS} = E\left[\sum_{i=1}^{p-1} \widehat{\sigma}_i^{2JS} (\widehat{\boldsymbol{\gamma}}_{(i)}^{JS} - \boldsymbol{\gamma}_{(i)})^\top \boldsymbol{\Sigma}_{(i+1)}^{-1} (\widehat{\boldsymbol{\gamma}}_{(i)}^{JS} - \boldsymbol{\gamma}_{(i)}) \right],$$

where the expectations are taken with respect to (7.31). Here, when $p \geq 4$, we consider improvement on

$$R_2^{JS} = E\left[\sum_{i=1}^{p-1} \widehat{\sigma}_i^{2JS} (p-i)/t_{i,i}^2 \right] = \sum_{i=1}^{p-1} (p-i) d_i^{JS}.$$

For $i = 1, \ldots, p-1$, denote $\boldsymbol{x}_{(i)} = \boldsymbol{t}_{(i)}/t_{i,i}$ and $\boldsymbol{S}_{(i)} = \boldsymbol{T}_{(i)}\boldsymbol{T}_{(i)}^\top$. Define

$$\widehat{\boldsymbol{\gamma}}_{(i)}^{SH} = \begin{cases} \left\{ 1 - \dfrac{p-i-2}{(n-p+3) t_{i,i}^2 \boldsymbol{x}_{(i)}^\top \boldsymbol{S}_{(i+1)}^{-1} \boldsymbol{x}_{(i)}} \right\} \boldsymbol{x}_{(i)} & \text{for } i = 1, \ldots, p-3, \\ \boldsymbol{x}_{(i)} & \text{for } i = p-2 \text{ and } p-1. \end{cases}$$

For $i = 1, \ldots, p-3$, $\widehat{\boldsymbol{\gamma}}_{(i)}^{SH}$ is the James-Stein (1961, Eq. 23) shrinkage estimator in estimation of the multivariate normal mean vector with unknown covariance matrix.

Note that $\boldsymbol{S}_{(i+1)} \sim \mathcal{W}_{p-i}(n-i, \boldsymbol{\Sigma}_{(i+1)})$ independent of $\boldsymbol{x}_{(i)}$ for each i. In a similar way to James and Stein (1961), we can show that for $i = 1, \ldots, p-3$

$$E\left[\widehat{\sigma}_i^{2JS}(\widehat{\boldsymbol{\gamma}}_{(i)}^{SH} - \boldsymbol{\gamma}_{(i)})^\top \boldsymbol{\Sigma}_{(i+1)}^{-1}(\widehat{\boldsymbol{\gamma}}_{(i)}^{SH} - \boldsymbol{\gamma}_{(i)})\right] \leq (p-i)d_i^{JS},$$

which implies that $\widehat{\boldsymbol{\Sigma}}^A$ obtained from using the $\widehat{\sigma}_i^{2JS}$'s and the $\widehat{\boldsymbol{\gamma}}_{(i)}^{SH}$'s dominates $\widehat{\boldsymbol{\Sigma}}^{JS}$ relative to the ordinary Stein loss (7.2).

For more details and improvement on R_1^{JS}, see Tsukuma (2014a, 2016b). The improvement on $\widehat{\boldsymbol{\Sigma}}^{JS}$ can also be done by using matricial shrinkage estimators of the mean matrix and this was discussed in Ma et al. (2012).

7.6.2 Decision-Theoretic Studies Under Quadratic Losses

Instead of the ordinary Stein loss (7.2) or the extended Stein loss (7.3), some quadratic-type loss functions have often been used for obtaining decision-theoretic results on covariance estimation. A typical quadratic loss is

$$L_1(\widehat{\boldsymbol{\Sigma}}, \boldsymbol{\Sigma}) = \operatorname{tr} \boldsymbol{\Sigma}^{-1}(\widehat{\boldsymbol{\Sigma}} - \boldsymbol{\Sigma})\boldsymbol{\Sigma}^{-1}(\widehat{\boldsymbol{\Sigma}} - \boldsymbol{\Sigma}) = \operatorname{tr} (\boldsymbol{\Sigma}^{-1}\widehat{\boldsymbol{\Sigma}} - \boldsymbol{I}_p)^2.$$

The L_1-loss is invariant under the general scale transformation $\boldsymbol{\Sigma} \to \boldsymbol{U}^\top \boldsymbol{\Sigma} \boldsymbol{U}$ and $\widehat{\boldsymbol{\Sigma}} \to \boldsymbol{U}^\top \widehat{\boldsymbol{\Sigma}} \boldsymbol{U}$ for any $\boldsymbol{U} \in \mathbb{U}_p$. Selliah (1964) addressed the $n \geq p$ case of covariance estimation under the L_1-loss and obtained a minimax estimator based on the Cholesky decomposition of the Wishart matrix. For other approaches, see Haff (1979b, 1980, 1991), Yang and Berger (1994) and Tsukuma (2014b). See also Konno (2009), who discussed the $p > n$ case under the L_1-loss.

A multivariate extension of squared error loss to covariance estimation may be defined by

$$L_2(\widehat{\boldsymbol{\Sigma}}, \boldsymbol{\Sigma}) = \operatorname{tr} (\widehat{\boldsymbol{\Sigma}} - \boldsymbol{\Sigma})^2,$$

namely, the squared Frobenius norm of $\widehat{\boldsymbol{\Sigma}} - \boldsymbol{\Sigma}$. The L_2-loss has orthogonal invariance under the orthogonal transformation $\boldsymbol{\Sigma} \to \boldsymbol{O}^\top \boldsymbol{\Sigma} \boldsymbol{O}$ and $\widehat{\boldsymbol{\Sigma}} \to \boldsymbol{O}^\top \widehat{\boldsymbol{\Sigma}} \boldsymbol{O}$ for any $\boldsymbol{O} \in \mathbb{O}_p$. In the literature, a much-discussed estimator is a linear shrinkage estimator $\widehat{\boldsymbol{\Sigma}}^{LS} = \alpha \widehat{\boldsymbol{\Sigma}}^{UB} + (1-\alpha)(\operatorname{tr} \widehat{\boldsymbol{\Sigma}}^{UB}/p)\boldsymbol{I}_p$, where $0 \leq \alpha \leq 1$ and $\widehat{\boldsymbol{\Sigma}}^{UB} = \boldsymbol{S}/n$ is the unbiased estimator of $\boldsymbol{\Sigma}$ under the normality assumption on error distribution. Leung and Chan (1998) suggested using $\alpha = n/(n+2)$ from a decision-theoretic point of view. This suggestion of Leung and Chan (1998) was extended to an elliptically contoured distribution model by Leung and Ng (2004). Ledoit and Wolf (2004) took an asymptotic approach to estimating an optimal α from sample under a general error distribution.

For $\mathbf{\Sigma} = (\sigma_{ij})$ and $\widehat{\mathbf{\Sigma}} = (\widehat{\sigma}_{ij})$, the L_2-loss can be generalized as

$$L_3(\widehat{\mathbf{\Sigma}}, \mathbf{\Sigma}) = \sum_{1 \le i \le j \le p} w_{ij}(\widehat{\sigma}_{ij} - \sigma_{ij})^2,$$

where $w_{ij} \ge 0$ for $1 \le i \le j \le p$. When $w_{ii} = 1$ for $i = 1, \ldots, p$ and $w_{ij} = 2$ for $1 \le i < j \le p$, the L_3-loss coincides with the L_2-loss. However, the L_3-loss does not includes the L_1-loss. For decision-theoretic results under the L_3-loss, see Perlman (1972) and Haff (1979b).

For $n \ge p$, as a variant type of the L_1-loss, we define

$$L_4(\widehat{\mathbf{\Sigma}}, \mathbf{\Sigma}) = \operatorname{tr} \widehat{\mathbf{\Sigma}}^{-1}(\widehat{\mathbf{\Sigma}} - \mathbf{\Sigma})\mathbf{\Sigma}^{-1}(\widehat{\mathbf{\Sigma}} - \mathbf{\Sigma}) = \operatorname{tr} \mathbf{\Sigma}^{-1}\widehat{\mathbf{\Sigma}} + \operatorname{tr} (\mathbf{\Sigma}^{-1}\widehat{\mathbf{\Sigma}})^{-1} - 2p.$$

The L_4-loss can also be obtained from the sum of the ordinary Stein loss (7.2) and its different entropy-type loss $L_P(\widehat{\mathbf{\Sigma}}, \mathbf{\Sigma}) = \operatorname{tr} (\mathbf{\Sigma}^{-1}\widehat{\mathbf{\Sigma}})^{-1} - \log |(\mathbf{\Sigma}^{-1}\widehat{\mathbf{\Sigma}})^{-1}| - p$. The invariance of the L_4-loss can easily be verified under a general scale transformation. Improved estimation under the L_4-loss was studied by Kubokawa and Konno (1990), Gupta and Ofori-Nyarko (1995) and Sun and Sun (2005).

7.6.3 Estimation of the Generalized Variance

Some statistical measures are formulated as functions of the covariance matrix. Generalized variance is the determinant of the covariance matrix and interpreted as a scalar measure of uncertainty.

Consider the case of $n \ge p$ in the model (7.1). The generalized variance is defined by $|\mathbf{\Sigma}|$. Denote an estimator of $|\mathbf{\Sigma}|$ by $|\widehat{\mathbf{\Sigma}}|$ and we now treat decision-theoretic estimation of $|\mathbf{\Sigma}|$ relative to a quadratic-type loss

$$L_G(|\widehat{\mathbf{\Sigma}}|, |\mathbf{\Sigma}|) = |\mathbf{\Sigma}|^{-2}(|\widehat{\mathbf{\Sigma}}| - |\mathbf{\Sigma}|)^2.$$

The Cholesky decomposition of $\boldsymbol{S}$ is denoted by $\boldsymbol{S} = \boldsymbol{T}\boldsymbol{T}^\top$, where $\boldsymbol{T} = (t_{ij}) \in \mathbb{L}_p^{(+)}$. Due to Proposition 3.10, it turns out that

$$E[|\boldsymbol{S}|] = \prod_{i=1}^{p} E[t_{ii}^2] = \prod_{i=1}^{p}(n - i + 1)\sigma_i^2 = |\mathbf{\Sigma}| \prod_{i=1}^{p}(n - i + 1),$$

so that

$$|\widehat{\mathbf{\Sigma}}^{UB}| = \left\{\prod_{i=1}^{p}(n - i + 1)^{-1}\right\} |\boldsymbol{S}| = \frac{(n - p + 2)!}{n!}|\boldsymbol{S}|$$

is the unbiased estimator of $|\boldsymbol{\Sigma}|$. However under the L_G-loss, $|\widehat{\boldsymbol{\Sigma}}^{UB}|$ is not the best among constant-multiple estimators of the form $c|\boldsymbol{S}|$ with positive constant c. The best constant c that minimizes risk of estimator $c|\boldsymbol{S}|$ is

$$c_0 = \frac{(n-p+2)!}{(n+2)!},$$

which can easily be verified by Proposition 3.10.

Here, any constant-multiple estimator $c|\boldsymbol{S}|$ is invariant under an affine transformation. Shorrock and Zidek (1976) discussed improvement on the best affine invariant estimator $|\widehat{\boldsymbol{\Sigma}}^{BC}| = c_0|\boldsymbol{S}|$ by using the information on $\boldsymbol{X}$. They showed that $|\widehat{\boldsymbol{\Sigma}}^{BC}|$ is dominated by

$$|\widehat{\boldsymbol{\Sigma}}^{SZ}| = \min\left\{\frac{(n-p+2)!}{(n+2)!}|\boldsymbol{S}|, \frac{(n+m-p+2)!}{(n+m+2)!}|\boldsymbol{S}+\boldsymbol{X}^\top\boldsymbol{X}|\right\}$$

relative to the L_G-loss. Clearly, the probability of $|\widehat{\boldsymbol{\Sigma}}^{SZ}| \le |\widehat{\boldsymbol{\Sigma}}^{BC}|$ is one, and hence $|\widehat{\boldsymbol{\Sigma}}^{SZ}|$ is shrinking $|\widehat{\boldsymbol{\Sigma}}^{BC}|$ toward the zero.

A different approach to proving the above dominance result is given by Sinha (1976). Rukhin and Sinha (1990) provided another dominance result without using the information on $\boldsymbol{X}$. Some results under an entropy-type loss are obtained by Sinha and Ghosh (1987) and Kubokawa and Srivastava (2003). On the other hand, a dominance result in the case of $p > n$ is still not known.

7.6.4 Estimation of the Precision Matrix

Assume now that $n \ge p$. Recall that $\boldsymbol{S} = \boldsymbol{Y}^\top\boldsymbol{Y} \sim \mathcal{W}_p(n, \boldsymbol{\Sigma})$. For any constant matrix $\boldsymbol{A} \in \mathbb{S}_p$, an application of the Haff identity (5.5) to $\operatorname{tr}\boldsymbol{\Sigma}^{-1}\boldsymbol{A}$ yields

$$\operatorname{tr}\boldsymbol{\Sigma}^{-1}\boldsymbol{A} = E[(n-p-1)\operatorname{tr}\boldsymbol{S}^{-1}\boldsymbol{A} + 2\operatorname{tr}\mathrm{D}_S\boldsymbol{A}] = E[(n-p-1)\operatorname{tr}\boldsymbol{S}^{-1}\boldsymbol{A}].$$

From the arbitrariness of $\boldsymbol{A}$, we obtain $\boldsymbol{\Sigma}^{-1} = E[(n-p-1)\boldsymbol{S}^{-1}]$, so that

$$\widehat{\boldsymbol{\Sigma}}^{-1}_{UB} = (n-p-1)\boldsymbol{S}^{-1}$$

is the unbiased estimator of $\boldsymbol{\Sigma}^{-1}$.

The inverse of the covariance matrix $\boldsymbol{\Sigma}$ is commonly called the precision matrix. The estimation problem of the precision matrix $\boldsymbol{\Sigma}^{-1}$ has been studied since Efron and Morris (1976). They pointed out that certain empirical Bayes estimation for a normal mean matrix is closely related to the problem of estimating $\boldsymbol{\Sigma}^{-1}$ under a quadratic-type loss

$$L_{EM}(\widehat{\boldsymbol{\Sigma}}^{-1}, \boldsymbol{\Sigma}^{-1}|\boldsymbol{S}) = \operatorname{tr}(\widehat{\boldsymbol{\Sigma}}^{-1} - \boldsymbol{\Sigma}^{-1})^2\boldsymbol{S}.$$

Here, we briefly introduce a unified approach to the $n \geq p$ and the $p > n$ cases based on the Efron-Morris (1976) estimator.

Let

$$\widehat{\boldsymbol{\Sigma}}_{BS}^{-1} = a_0 \boldsymbol{S}^{+}, \quad a_0 = |n - p| - 1.$$

Among estimators of the form $a\boldsymbol{S}^{+}$ with positive constant a, $\widehat{\boldsymbol{\Sigma}}_{BS}^{-1}$ is the best estimator relative to the L_{EM}-loss, and, when $n \geq p$, $\widehat{\boldsymbol{\Sigma}}_{BS}^{-1}$ is equivalent to $\widehat{\boldsymbol{\Sigma}}_{UB}^{-1}$. To improve $\widehat{\boldsymbol{\Sigma}}_{BS}^{-1}$, we define the Efron-Morris (1976) type estimator as

$$\widehat{\boldsymbol{\Sigma}}_{EM}^{-1} = \widehat{\boldsymbol{\Sigma}}_{BS}^{-1} + \frac{(\nu - 1)(\nu + 2)}{\operatorname{tr} \boldsymbol{S}} \boldsymbol{S}\boldsymbol{S}^{+}$$

with $\nu = n \wedge p$. If $n \geq p$, then $\widehat{\boldsymbol{\Sigma}}_{EM}^{-1}$ is the same as in Efron and Morris (1976). Denote by $\boldsymbol{S} = \boldsymbol{H}\boldsymbol{L}\boldsymbol{H}^{\top}$ the eigenvalue decomposition of $\boldsymbol{S}$, where $\boldsymbol{L} \in \mathbb{D}_{\nu}^{(\geq 0)}$ and $\boldsymbol{H} \in \mathbb{V}_{p,\nu}$, and then note that

$$\widehat{\boldsymbol{\Sigma}}_{EM}^{-1} = \boldsymbol{H}\boldsymbol{\Phi}^{EM}\boldsymbol{H}^{\top}, \quad \boldsymbol{\Phi}^{EM} = a_0 \boldsymbol{L}^{-1} + \frac{(\nu - 1)(\nu + 2)}{\operatorname{tr} \boldsymbol{L}} \boldsymbol{I}_{\nu}.$$

Proposition 7.11 *$\widehat{\boldsymbol{\Sigma}}_{EM}^{-1}$ dominates $\widehat{\boldsymbol{\Sigma}}_{BS}^{-1}$ relative to the L_{EM}-loss.*

The proof of Proposition 7.11 can be provided by an unbiased risk estimate method and it is omitted.

For decision-theoretic estimation of the precision matrix with $n \geq p$, other procedures for improving the unbiased estimator can be found in Haff (1977, 1979a, b), Dey (1987) and Dey et al. (1990). An improving method via using information on means was considered by Sinha and Ghosh (1987). Eaton and Olkin (1987) and Krishnamoorthy and Gupta (1989) provided minimax estimators based on the Cholesky decomposition of the Wishart matrix $\boldsymbol{S}$ relative to the Stein-type loss

$$L_P(\widehat{\boldsymbol{\Sigma}}^{-1}, \boldsymbol{\Sigma}^{-1}) = \operatorname{tr} \boldsymbol{\Sigma}\widehat{\boldsymbol{\Sigma}}^{-1} - \log |\boldsymbol{\Sigma}\widehat{\boldsymbol{\Sigma}}^{-1}| - p.$$

See also Zhou et al. (2001) and Tsukuma (2014b) for related works to improved minimax estimation. Orthogonally invariant minimax estimators are obtained by Perron (1997) and Kubokawa (2005) for $p = 2$ and by Sheena (2003) for $p = 3$. However, for $p \geq 4$, orthogonally invariant minimax estimators are still not provided.

The $p > n$ case is treated by Kubokawa and Srivastava (2008), who propose some improved estimators under quadratic-type losses.

References

D.K. Dey, Improved estimation of a multinormal precision matrix. Stat. Probab. Lett. **6**, 125–128 (1987)

D.K. Dey, M. Ghosh, C. Srinivasan, A new class of improved estimators of a multinormal precision matrix. Stat. Decisions **8**, 141–151 (1990)

D.K. Dey, C. Srinivasan, Estimation of a covariance matrix under Stein's loss. Ann. Stat. **13**, 1581–1591 (1985)

M.L. Eaton. Some problems in covariance estimation. Technical Reports No. 49, (Department of Statistics, Stanford University, 1970)

M.L. Eaton, I. Olkin, Best equivariant estimators of a Cholesky decomposition. Ann. Stat. **15**, 1639–1650 (1987)

B. Efron, C. Morris, Multivariate empirical Bayes and estimation of covariance matrices. Ann. Stat. **4**, 22–32 (1976)

A.K. Gupta, S. Ofori-Nyarko, Improved minimax estimators of normal covariance and precision matrices. Statistics **26**, 19–25 (1995)

L.R. Haff, Minimax estimators for a multinormal precision matrix. J. Multivar. Anal. **7**, 374–385 (1977)

L.R. Haff, Estimation of the inverse covariance matrix: Random mixtures of the inverse Wishart matrix and the identity. Ann. Stat. **7**, 1264–1276 (1979a)

L.R. Haff, An identity for the Wishart distribution with applications. J. Multivar. Anal. **9**, 531–544 (1979b)

L.R. Haff, Empirical Bayes estimation of the multivariate normal covariance matrix. Ann. Stat. **8**, 586–597 (1980)

L.R. Haff, The variational form of certain Bayes estimators. Ann. Stat. **19**, 1163–1190 (1991)

W. James, C. Stein, Estimation with quadratic loss, in *Proceedings of the Fourth Berkeley Symposium on Mathematical Statistics and Probability*, vol. 1, ed. by J. Neyman, (University of California Press, Berkeley, 1961),pp. 361–379

J. Kiefer, Invariance, minimax sequential estimation, and continuous time processes. Ann. Math. Stat. **28**, 573–601 (1957)

Y. Konno, Shrinkage estimators for large covariance matrices in multivariate real and complex normal distributions under an invariant quadratic loss. J. Multivar. Anal. **100**, 2237–2253 (2009)

K. Krishnamoorthy, A.K. Gupta, Improved minimax estimation of a normal precision matrix. Can. J. Stat. **17**, 91–102 (1989)

T. Kubokawa, A revisit to estimating of the precision matrix of the Wishart distribution. J. Stat. Res. **39**, 91–114 (2005)

T. Kubokawa, Y. Konno, Estimating the covariance matrix and the generalized variance under a symmetric loss. Ann. Inst. Stat. Math. **42**, 331–343 (1990)

T. Kubokawa, C. Robert, AKMdE Saleh, Empirical Bayes estimation of the variance parameter of a normal distribution with unknown mean under an entropy loss. Sankhyā Ser. A **54**, 402–410 (1992)

T. Kubokawa, M.S. Srivastava, Estimating the covariance matrix: a new approach. J. Multivar. Anal. **86**, 28–47 (2003)

T. Kubokawa, M.S. Srivastava, Estimation of the precision matrix of a singular Wishart distribution and its application in high-dimensional data. J. Multivar. Anal. **99**, 1906–1928 (2008)

T. Kubokawa, M.-T. Tsai, Estimation of covariance matrices in fixed and mixed effects linear models. J. Multivar. Anal. **97**, 2242–2261 (2006)

O. Ledoit, M. Wolf, A well-conditioned estimator for large-dimensional covariance matrices. J. Multivar. Anal. **88**, 365–411 (2004)

P.L. Leung, W.Y. Chan, Estimation of the scale matrix and its eigenvalues in the Wishart and the multivariate F distributions. Ann. Inst. Stat. Math. **50**, 523–530 (1998)

P.L. Leung, F.Y. Ng, Improved estimation of a covariance matrix in an elliptically contoured matrix distribution. J. Multivar. Anal. **88**, 131–137 (2004)
S.P. Lin, M.D. Perlman, A monte carlo comparison of four estimators for a covariance matrix, in *Multivar. Anal. VI*, ed. by P.R. Krishnaiah (North-Holland, Amsterdam, 1985), pp. 411–429
T. Ma, L. Jia, Y. Su, A new estimator of covariance matrix. J. Stat. Plan. Infer. **142**, 529–536 (2012)
M.D. Perlman, Reduced mean square error estimation for several parameters. Sankhyā Ser. B **34**, 89–92 (1972)
F. Perron, Equivariant estimators of the covariance matrix. Can. J. Stat. **18**, 179–182 (1990)
F. Perron, Minimax estimators of a covariance matrix. J. Multivar. Anal. **43**, 16–28 (1992)
F. Perron, On a conjecture of Krishnamoorthy and Gupta. J. Multivar. Anal. **62**, 110–120 (1997)
T. Robertson, F.T. Wright, R.L. Dykstra, *Order Restricted Statistical Inference* (Wiley, New York, 1988)
A.L. Rukhin, B.K. Sinha, Decision-theoretic estimation of the product of gamma scales and generalized variance. Calcutta Stat. Assoc. Bull. **40**, 257–265 (1990)
D. Sharma, K. Krishnamoorthy, Orthogonal equivariant minimax estimators of bivariate normal covariance matrix and precision matrix. Calcutta Stat. Assoc. Bull. **32**, 23–46 (1983)
J.B. Selliah, Estimation and testing problems in a Wishart distribution. Technical reports No.10 (Department of Statistics, Stanford University, 1964)
Y. Sheena, On minimaxity of the normal precision matrix estimator of Krishnamoorthy and Gupta. Statistics **37**, 387–399 (2003)
Y. Sheena, A. Takemura, Inadmissibility of non-order-preserving orthogonally invariant estimators of the covariance matrix in the case of Stein's loss. J. Multivar. Anal. **41**, 117–131 (1992)
R.B. Shorrock, J.V. Zidek, An improved estimator of the generalized variance. Ann. Stat. **4**, 629–638 (1976)
B.K. Sinha, On improved estimators of the generalized variance. J. Multivar. Anal. **6**, 617–626 (1976)
B.K. Sinha, M. Ghosh, Inadmissibility of the best equivariant estimators of the variance-covariance matrix, the precision matrix, and the generalized variance under entropy loss. Stat. Dec. **5**, 201–227 (1987)
C. Stein, Some problems in multivariate analysis, Part I. Technical Reports No.6 (Department of Statistics, Stanford University, 1956)
C. Stein, Inadmissibility of the usual estimator for the variance of a normal distribution with unknown mean. Ann. Inst. Stat. Math. **16**, 155–160 (1964)
C. Stein, *Estimation of a Covariance Matrix, Rietz Lecture, 39th Annual Meeting IMS* (Atlanta, GA, 1975)
C. Stein, Lectures on the theory of estimation of many parameters, in *Proceedings of Scientific Seminars of the Steklov Institute Studies in the Statistical Theory of Estimation, Part I*, vol. 74, eds. by I.A. Ibragimov, M.S. Nikulin (Leningrad Division, 1977), pp. 4–65
W.E. Strawderman, Minimaxity. J. Am. Stat. Assoc. **95**, 1364–1368 (2000)
D. Sun, X. Sun, Estimation of the multivariate normal precision and covariance matrices in a star-shape model. Ann. Inst. Stat. Math. **57**, 455–484 (2005)
A. Takemura, An orthogonally invariant minimax estimator of the covariance matrix of a multivariate normal population. Tsukuba J. Math. **8**, 367–376 (1984)
H. Tsukuma, Minimax covariance estimation using commutator subgroup of lower triangular matrices. J. Multivar. Anal. **124**, 333–344 (2014a)
H. Tsukuma, Improvement on the best invariant estimators of the normal covariance and precision matrices via a lower triangular subgroup. J. Jpn. Stat. Soc. **44**, 195–218 (2014b)
H. Tsukuma, Estimation of a high-dimensional covariance matrix with the Stein loss. J. Multivar. Anal. **148**, 1–17 (2016a)
H. Tsukuma, Minimax estimation of a normal covariance matrix with the partial Iwasawa decomposition. J. Multivar. Anal. **145**, 190–207 (2016b)
H. Tsukuma, T. Kubokawa, Minimaxity in estimation of restricted and non-restricted scale parameter matrices. Ann. Inst. Stat. Math. **67**, 261–285 (2015)

H. Tsukuma, T. Kubokawa, Unified improvements in estimation of a normal covariance matrix in high and low dimensions. J. Multivar. Anal. **143**, 233–248 (2016)

R. Yang, J.O. Berger, Estimation of a covariance matrix using the reference prior. Ann. Stat. **22**, 1195–1211 (1994)

X. Zhou, X. Sun, J. Wang, Estimation of the multivariate normal precision matrix under the entropy loss. Ann. Inst. Stat. Math. **53**, 760–768 (2001)

Index

H. Tsukuma and T. Kubokawa, *Shrinkage Estimation for Mean and Covariance Matrices*, JSS Research Series in Statistics, https://doi.org/10.1007/978-981-15-1596-5

Printed in the United States
By Bookmasters

Printed in the United States
By Bookmasters